A Patient Safety Handbook for

AMBULATORY CARE
PROVIDERS

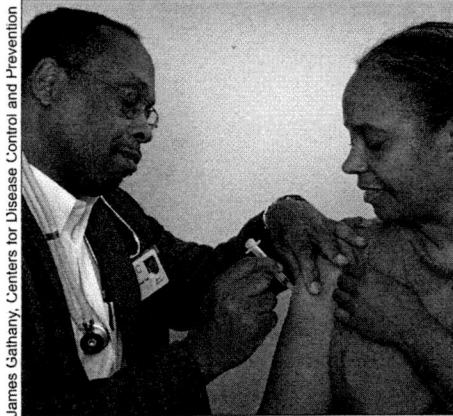

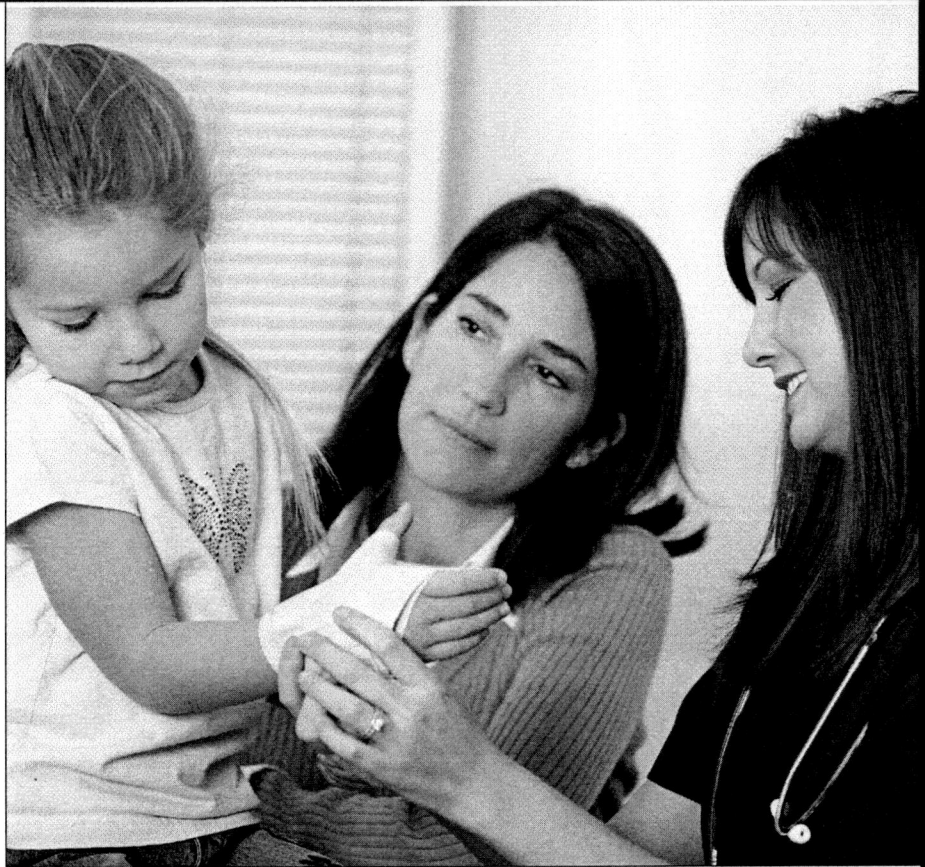

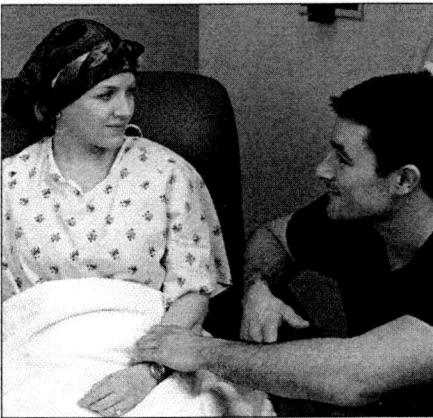

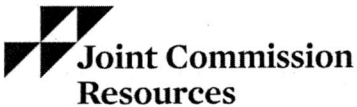

MW01528249

Joint Commission Resources

Senior Editor: Helen M. Fry
Senior Project Manager: Cheryl Firestone
Associate Director, Production: Johanna Harris
Associate Director, Editorial Development: Diane Bell
Executive Director: Catherine Chopp Hinckley, Ph.D.
Joint Commission/JCR Reviewers: Michael Kulczycki, Beverley Robins, Lon Berkeley, Virginia McCollum, Joyce Webb, Deborah Nadzam, Michael Jarema, Diane Bell

Joint Commission Resources Mission

The mission of Joint Commission Resources is to continuously improve the safety and quality of care in the United States and in the international community through the provision of education and consultation services and international accreditation.

Joint Commission Resources educational programs and publications support, but are separate from, the accreditation activities of The Joint Commission. Attendees at Joint Commission Resources educational programs and purchasers of Joint Commission Resources publications receive no special consideration or treatment in, or confidential information about, the accreditation process.

The inclusion of an organization name, product, or service in a Joint Commission publication should not be construed as an endorsement of such organization, product, or service, nor is failure to include an organization name, product, or service to be construed as disapproval.

Printed in the U.S.A. 5 4 3 2 1

Requests for permission to make copies of any part of this work should be mailed to
Permissions Editor
Department of Publications
Joint Commission Resources
One Renaissance Boulevard
Oakbrook Terrace, Illinois 60181
permissions@jcrinc.com

ISBN: 978-1-59940-367-0
Library of Congress Control Number: 2009933248

For more information about Joint Commission Resources, please visit http://www.jcrinc.com.

Contents

How Safe Are Your Patients?

Ambulatory care organizations face critical patient safety issues, as do hospitals and other inpatient health care settings. These issues include ensuring medication safety, preventing infections, meeting challenges with the facility environment, and communicating effectively with patients and with other providers and departments.

Because ambulatory surgical centers, office-based surgery practices, community health centers, diagnostic imaging centers, urgent care centers, medical and dental centers, and other ambulatory care facilities provide ambulatory care only, they face unique patient safety issues and possess a different set of strengths and challenges for tackling these issues.

Providing a safe environment for patients to receive health care is a universal concern. Several different organizations and agencies—federal, state, and private—have addressed the many interlocking components of patient safety with the ultimate goal of eliminating error, standardizing protocols, and involving all stakeholders in solutions and policies. Still, health care errors are a leading cause of patient injury and death throughout the United States.[1,2] How well are we doing in meeting our goals?

As compared with inpatient and other settings for health care delivery, errors in ambulatory health care (AHC) settings may appear to be less significant per error; but in the aggregate and over time, they may cause greater harm.[3] Because hospitals, rather than ambulatory settings, have been the major focus of safety initiatives, the data are not as often available, and therefore the consequences of errors in AHC may not be recognized as quickly. Identifying and implementing solutions to prevent further errors may be more of a challenge.

Researchers at the Feinberg School of Medicine of Northwestern University concluded that the ambulatory setting can be a "risky context of care that leads to hospital admission, injury, and death."[4] The findings were based on a 2007 analysis of the Colorado and Utah Medical Practices Study, which reviewed adverse events and preventable adverse events that occurred in an ambulatory setting and resulted in a hospital admission.

Their findings showed that annually in the United States, an estimated 75,000 hospitalizations are related to preventable adverse events occurring in the ambulatory setting. A total of 10% of these cases resulted in serious permanent injury (n = 4,839) or death (n = 2,587).

Estimates of error rates in ambulatory care settings may be low because errors are sometimes harder to catch. There are a few reasons for this:

- The patient is a moving target. By virtue of the environment, the patient has walked out the door after a short interaction, sometimes as little as 10 to 15 minutes.
- AHC can involve complex care provided in a variety of settings by a variety of providers.
- The patient safety movement is riddled with a lack of consensus about what constitutes an error, both in the medical literature and in the thinking of some clinicians,[5] and even within some individual medical practices, a lack of clear definitions and varied interpretations may influence the identification and reporting of errors.

For instance, which of the scenarios in Sidebar 1, page vi, would you consider an error?

The study from which these five clinical scenarios were drawn was begun as a systematic literature review.[5] A survey including these scenarios was sent to members of the American Academy of Family Physicians, and to a panel of experts, to query whether an error had occurred. The pilot survey results were analyzed qualitatively to search for insights into what may affect the use of the term *error*. Although the definition originated by James Reason predominated the literature search, the researchers found 25 different definitions for *error* in the medical literature. The authors concluded that three areas may affect how physicians make decisions about *error*: the process that occurred versus the outcome that occurred, rare versus common occurrences, and system versus individual responsibility.

From the study results, the authors generated a model proposing three additional elements important to making a decision about whether an event is an error.[5] These elements are to ask the following questions:

Sidebar 1. Clinical Scenarios Used in a Survey of Family Physicians

Which of the following do you consider a medical error?

1. Dr. Jones ordered liver function tests to evaluate Mr. Black's health complaints. The next day, a report of Mr. Black's lipids (but not liver function tests) shows up on Dr. Jones's desk, and the results were within normal range. Dr. Jones documented "normal lipids, notify patient" and sent it to his nurse. A week later, Mr. Black returned, more ill, and was found to have acute hepatitis A.

2. Mrs. Rose, a patient with high blood pressure, had a basic metabolic profile performed, and was found to have a random blood glucose of 189. Dr. Smith documented "have patient return for repeat glucose and glycohemoglobin." The nurse documented "attempted phone call, no answer." Eight months later, the patient returned with a yeast infection and was found to have a random blood glucose of 356, which is significantly higher than normal range.

3. Dr. Miller reviewed a large number of lab results from his "normal lab results" folder and sent them to be filed. The next month he saw Ms. Brown again for menstrual irregularities. In reviewing her chart, Dr. Miller saw that he wrote "normal, ok to file" next to an elevated TSH of 37 (normal range = 0.4 to 4.5 mIU/L).

4. Mr. White had blood drawn by Dr. Jones's medical assistant for an ordered test. After he left, she dropped the tube and broke it. Mr. White was called, and he made another visit to the office to get his blood drawn the next day.

5. Ms. Green wanted to know the results of a computed tomography (CT) head scan ordered by her physician to evaluate her headaches. The test had been performed the previous week at the hospital radiology department routinely used by the ambulatory care clinic. Ms. Green called the office and left a message asking the physician or nurse to call her. When no one returned her call, she called back two days later and made an appointment. At the visit, the CT results were not in her chart and could not be found in the office.

Source: Modified from Elder N.C., Pallerla H., Regan S.: What do family physicians consider an error? A comparison of definitions and physician perception. *BMC Fam Pract* 7:73, Dec. 8, 2006.

1. Do I know the outcome, and is there harm from this event?
2. Is this event a common or rare occurrence?
3. Does the responsibility for this event lie predominantly with an individual or with the system?

These three questions are useful when assessing an AHC climate and specific issues at hand.

Before delving into the particulars of safety maintenance and error prevention, it is advantageous to consider how safety initiatives make good business sense.

The Business Case for Patient Safety

In addition to the mandate to provide the highest-quality and safest care, investing in patient safety makes good business sense. Safety violations cost money, resources, and time; in contrast, safety initiatives reduce resource spending. Thus, implementing initiatives brings a high return on investment from a decreased cost of errors, an increased level of patient satisfaction (referrals and loyal patients help increase volumes), an increased level of staff satisfaction (decreased turnover, better care), and a shift toward more ambulatory care in the industry (with ambulatory care pay-for-performance likely to be on the horizon, this may mean greater future reimbursements).[6] There are many organizational benefits of investing in patient safety initiatives, as presented in Table 1, page vii.

After an organization commits to safety excellence, as mentioned previously, a next step is to set clear definitions of terms so that when identifying and improving systems and processes, all staff are viewing safety from within the same paradigm.

Medical Errors Defined

Numerous definitions and terms for *medical error* are used in the literature. For purposes of our discussions in this book, we define *medical error* according to the widely accepted definition used by James Reason: "Medical error is the failure of planned actions to achieve their desired goal."[7] A *near miss* (close call, almost error) is defined as "any process variation that did not affect an outcome but for which a recurrence carries a significant chance of a serious adverse outcome."[7] A *sentinel event* is defined by The Joint Commission as an unexpected occurrence involving death or serious physical or psychological injury, or the

Table 1. Organizational Benefits of Investing in Patient Safety Initiatives		
Areas	**Impact of Patient Safety Lapses**	**Impact of Patient Safety Initiatives**
Financial	• Decreased profit margins • Increased direct and indirect costs • Threat to organizational survival	• Decreased costs • Prepared for pay-for-performance • Increased capacity and infrastructure
Clinical	• Compromised quality of care • Reduced organizational performance • Promotes variability in service delivery • Increased inappropriate care • Costly duplication of services	• Improved clinical quality indicators • Increased adherence to care guidelines • Provides better patient care • Increased workflow efficiencies • Enhanced process design
Technological	• Illegible and incomplete orders • Increased potential for errors due to use of paper chart • Records availability problems	• Decreased medication errors • Supports coordinated care management • Optimized access to clinical data • Increased ability for electronic ordering
Culture	• Promotes a "blame" culture • Increased fear of error disclosure	• Fosters a culture of safety • Maximizes error interception
Legal	• Consumes additional resources pursuing litigation defense, paying settlements and awards	• Avoids exposure to liability • Increased documentation accuracy • Reduced insurance premiums
Legislation/ Regulation	• Potential sanctions and litigation	• Complies with patient safety standards
Human Resources	• Increased recruitment costs of scarce human resources • Compromised employee morale • Reduced patient and family satisfaction	• Increased provider and patient satisfaction • Increased provider-patient communication • Higher productivity with efficient process • Eases provider recruitment
Measurement	• Threatens transparency and accountability • Reduced provider and system feedback • Delays patient safety improvement • May compromise HIPAA requirements	• Enhanced surveillance and monitoring • Prepared for public reporting • Enhanced benchmarking and goal settings • Increased patient confidentiality
Marketing	• Tarnished reputation and brand identity • Decreased public confidence • Decreases new business initiatives	• Builds good will and reputation • Elevated brand image and differentiation • Increased revenue by bringing new patients
Accreditation Stakeholders	• Increased regulatory costs • Duplication of efforts and messages • Uncoordinated safety requirements	• If accredited, maintains accreditation • Simplifies HIPAA compliance • Aligns with other organizations

Source: Adapted from Sabogal F., Snow A., Sawyer L.: The business case for patient safety. *CAHQ Journal* 32:10–16, 27–34, Jan.–Mar. 2008.

risk thereof. Serious injury specifically includes loss of limb or function. The phrase "or the risk thereof" includes any process variation for which a recurrence would carry a significant chance of a serious adverse outcome. Such events are called "sentinel" because they signal the need for immediate investigation and response.[8]

To truly grasp the significance of adopting a culture

of safety within an organization, it is important to examine the effect of errors in AHC.

Ambulatory-Specific Statistics on Errors

Little research has been done to date to identify and catalog patient safety initiatives and recommendations outside the hospital setting. Thanks to work by the National Quality Forum, Utilization Review Accreditation Commitee, National Committee on

Quality Assurance, and The Joint Commission, interest and awareness has been raised on the importance of patient safety in the ambulatory and home settings.[9] The following are some of the findings:

- Between 1995 and 2004, the number of outpatient visits rose from 414 million to 571 million.[10] As the lengths of stay in hospitals have decreased over the past decade, the total number of outpatient care delivery visits has risen.
- Out of every seven outpatient care visits, one includes a medical error of some kind.[3]
- Of those errors, 24% result in harm and 70% have the potential to cause harm.[3]
- As noted in a 2006 report from the Institute of Medicine, approximately 530,000 Medicare beneficiaries in ambulatory care clinics experienced a medication-related error in the year.[11]
- In a study limited to AHC, 59% of all settled malpractice claims involved diagnostic errors that caused patient harm.[12]
- The five major causes of medical errors in primary care are ordering medications, implementing lab tests, filing system errors, dispensing medications, and responding to abnormal lab test results.[11]

How the Ambulatory Environment Differs from the Hospital Setting

Understanding the nature and effect of ambulatory care risks can help direct attention toward targets for improving patient safety. In many respects, ambulatory and hospital environments share both similarities and differences. But the opportunities for error and associated injuries are likely to differ from hospital-based care by type of ambulatory setting, type of care (for example, diagnostic, surgery), and population (age group, ethnic or racial groups).[4]

Challenges in Ambulatory Health Care

In ambulatory care, a number of challenges differ from those faced in an inpatient setting, mainly staff skill mix, fewer support staff, and budget limitations. Particular challenges that ambulatory care organizations face include the following:

- There are often fewer resources, such as staff and funds, which can impact physician and staff performance. In one survey, 48% of family physicians and internists considered their practices chaotic.[3] Sixty-one percent said they were stressed out, and more than 25% said they were burned out.

- In hospitals, quality improvement and safety officers are available; in ambulatory settings you often have only the physician and nursing staff.[13,14]
- Staff are multitasking and responsible for a broader range of areas.
- Ensuring continuity of care can be more challenging due to the frequent use of off-site laboratory and pharmacy services and specialty providers.[4]
- Patients in the ambulatory setting are often primarily responsible for coordinating their own care.[4]
- Patients in ambulatory care may be their own source of safety risks (infection, unsafe practices).[14]
- The patient is a moving target; communication/transition issues may be more challenging.[14]
- Distractions of an ambulatory or office setting include phones, time restraints, and large visit schedules.
- An increasing complexity of patients exists, particularly from chronic illness.
- Staff have differing skill levels and may have limited scope of knowledge related to the risk of harm from seemingly small mistakes.
- Staff may have less experience with performance improvement tasks such as data collection and analysis and other components of performance improvement.
- Regulatory forces are typically less active in ambulatory care.

Opportunities in Ambulatory Health Care

Conversely, as compared to inpatient care, many unique opportunities for improving safety in ambulatory care exist:

- Patients may not be as acutely ill and may be better able to provide self-care.
- Patients may be more easily engaged in their own care, which can support a patient-centric system of care.
- A shift to increase research for safety initiatives in AHC means the availability of new tools and methods are also rapidly increasing.
- A smaller environment and fewer staff can enable communication, providing an opportunity to more quickly implement new policies in the organization.
- Fewer staff can also mean a greater sense of teamwork to reduce the impact of a "blame and shame" culture environment.
- Interventions may include a simple educational tool or system redesign that can require limited commitment of time and money and may be easier to institute in an AHC system.

How The Joint Commission Can Help

One of the key elements of The Joint Commission's commitment to patient safety is its ongoing focus on safety-related standards.[15] The standards include requirements to maintain safety systemwide and thus provide a structure for patient safety efforts. Joint Commission requirements include safety as a focus, leadership guidelines, and the National Patient Safety Goals.

Priority Focus Area: Patient Safety

Almost all of The Joint Commission standards are related to safety and quality issues. Although safety considerations have always been included in The Joint Commission requirements, each revision brings these issues to the forefront of leadership, staff, and patient and family awareness.

Leadership Standards

Joint Commission Leadership standards address the level to which a facility or institution reports, investigates, and documents its organizational problems and failures. In particular, an emphasis is placed on the leader's responsibility to encourage a workplace environment that recognizes the importance of safety. The Leadership standards describe the leader's role in a comprehensive safety program. These standards do the following[15]:

- Encourage decision making as a collaborative activity
- Require organizations to implement an integrated patient safety program throughout the organization
- Ensure that processes are well designed and incorporate available information from internal as well as external sources
- Require organization leaders to adequately allocate human, information, time, physical, and financial resources to support activities
- Measure and assess leadership contributions to performance and patient safety

Value of the National Patient Safety Goals to Ambulatory Health Care Organizations

The National Patient Safety Goals can help health care organizations focus attention and resources on the work of maintaining patient safety. The goals are available at The Joint Commission Web site: http://www.jointcommission.org/PatientSafety/NationalPatientSafetyGoals/. One of the areas that has received particular attention is that of sentinel events.

Sentinel Events. The Joint Commission has worked diligently with health care organizations to conduct risk assessment and root cause analysis (RCA) and construct means to prevent and avoid sentinel events. The Joint Commission Sentinel Event Policy requires that any time a sentinel event occurs, health care organizations must complete a thorough and credible RCA, implement improvements to reduce risk, and monitor the effectiveness of those improvements.[15] The policy also encourages organizations to report to The Joint Commission any sentinel events that resulted in death or serious injury, along with their root causes and related preventive actions. This facilitates The Joint Commission, sharing lessons learned with other health care organizations to prevent like recurrences of similar events. Although these reporting systems may be more entrenched in inpatient situations, AHC organizations can also benefit from reporting sentinel events in the ambulatory setting.

For example, in a *Sentinel Event Alert* issued in April 2008 regarding pediatric medication errors, The Joint Commission issued suggestions for preventive actions to be taken in ambulatory (as well as inpatient) settings, including effective medication standardization and identification and judicious use of technology.[16] A September 2008 *Alert* on anticoagulation errors included Joint Commission suggested actions for heparin orders in the outpatient setting.[17]

In its ongoing work, The Joint Commission addresses the potential reduction of goals to further enable the focus on improving patient safety.

About This Book

Ambulatory care organizations require a different set of strategies for keeping patients safe in their setting. However, almost all patient safety benchmarks and improvement initiatives available today specifically target hospitals and may not directly translate to the ambulatory care setting.

Tight schedules, an increased focus on productivity and throughput, and limited budgets leave little time and fewer resources for safety projects and staff training. Still, your patients expect your organization to provide safe, quality care and prevent harm from reaching them. You need a resource that provides proven solutions for keeping your patients safe in an ambulatory setting. *A*

Patient Safety Handbook for Ambulatory Health Care Providers addresses the challenging patient safety concerns you face on a daily basis in your ambulatory care setting and was developed specifically for this setting. Particular emphasis is given to the National Patient Safety Goals that increased in depth or scope, and to the goals for which organizational noncompliance increased over the past few years. These may be areas in which barriers and contributing factors stand in the way of compliance, and patients therefore face higher risk. These areas include reporting critical test results, labeling medications and solutions, hand hygiene guidelines, medication reconciliation, and conducting a time-out process before a surgical procedure.

The book is organized according to system-level issues to help you find what you need fast. It also contains useful tools that educate staff and physicians about patient safety in ambulatory care:

- Easy-to-adapt forms, checklists, and solutions
- Critical lessons learned about which approaches work, which don't, and why
- Real-life case studies on improving patient safety in ambulatory settings
- Helpful boxes that define key terms, identify Joint Commission requirements, or explain targeted performance improvement tools

It should be noted that the tools featured in these chapters may be applicable to more than just the topic area in which they are first located. Our goal was to identify tools and examples strictly from the pool of freestanding ambulatory care organizations. However, in some cases the best information available originated from hospital-based ambulatory care. This information can be directly applicable or easily modified for AHC.

This book explores seven essential areas. A chapter-by-chapter description follows.

- Chapter 1, "Patient-Centered Care." This chapter defines patient-centered care and where this concept plays out in particular safety areas in AHC. Patients' involvement with their own care is integral to providing extra safeguards to prevent errors.

- Chapter 2, "Communication." This chapter shows how communication plays a role in maintaining safety in ambulatory care. Techniques and tools are provided to assist in improving staff communication skills and to examine the particular areas in which communication breakdowns can increase safety risks, including errors involving filing systems, transitions of care, and telephone and other verbal orders.

- Chapter 3, "Medication Use." This chapter discusses the various ways that storing, dispensing, and administering medications, and coordinating communications regarding medication use, may pose risks to patient safety. The text provides solutions for preventing medication errors and improving those communications between providers and patients.

- Chapter 4, "Surgical Safety." This chapter discusses patient safety during surgical procedures and anesthesia administration and aspects of monitoring patient recovery. Preparedness for emergency and disaster events, such as patient burns and surgical fires, is also addressed. Preventive practices for reducing surgical site infections are provided, and tools such as checklists are provided for assessment of wrong-site surgery and The Joint Commission Universal Protocol.

- Chapter 5, "Infection Prevention and Control." This chapter discusses best practices for infection prevention in the ambulatory setting, including hand hygiene; infection-related sentinel events; and tracking data, including outcomes data.

- Chapter 6, "Environment and Equipment." This chapter discusses topics relevant to environmental and equipment-related issues that may pose risks to patient (and staff) safety. This includes emergency management plans, sterilization efforts, safety using radiation and in imaging, and workflow redesign. Patient safety rounds are addressed as a means of identifying safety issues. Safe practices for magnetic resonance imaging and radiation, and the use of patient tracers in the ambulatory surgical suite, are also discussed.

- Chapter 7, "Staff Education and Training." This chapter discusses the most crucial areas for staff safety training, including requirements in credentialing and orientation, and specific topics for training: performance improvement, performing patient assessments, performing mobile lifts and transport safety to and from the ambulatory surgical center, aseptic technique and sterilization monitoring, moderate sedation safety, fire safety, and teamwork considerations.

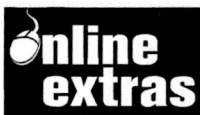

online extras In addition to the material in this book, bonus Online Extras can be found at http://www.jcrinc.com/PSAC09/extras/.

Acknowledgements

We would like to thank the individuals, institutions, and organizations that contributed information for this book. We are particularly grateful to the many people who contributed their time and information to construct the case studies:

- Lisa Petrusky, R.N., Manager, Quality Assurance, American Access Care, Monongahela, PA

- Lisa Faller, R.N., C.A.S.C., Director of Quality, American Access Care, Orlando, FL

- Linda Massaro, Director, Quality Improvement, InSight Health Corp., Wexford, PA

- Sheila M. Warren M.P.H., R.N., C.P.H.Q., Patient Safety Consultant, WebCident Patient Safety Administrator, Indian Health Service–Headquarters, Rockville, MD

- CDR Lawrence M. Zubel, O.D., Chief of Optometry, Performance Improvement Committee Chair, Phoenix Area Indian Health Service, Ft. Duchesne, UT

- Heather Huentelman, Pharm.D., HIV Clinical Pharmacist, Phoenix Indian Medical Center, Phoenix

- Stephen A. Maurer, Pharm.D., Chief Pharmacist, Phoenix Indian Medical Center, Phoenix

- Milton "Mickey" Eder, Ph.D., Director of Research Programs, Access Community Health Network, Chicago

- Nancy Elder, M.D., M.S.P.H., Department of Family Medicine, University of Cincinnati, Cincinnati

- John Hickner, M.D., M.Sc., The University of Chicago Pritzker School of Medicine, Professor of Family Medicine, University of Chicago

- Sandy G. Smith, Ph.D., Senior Education Specialist, Pritzker School of Medicine, The University of Chicago

- Dianne Daugherty, Executive Director, Malignant Hyperthermia Association of the United States, Sherburne, NY

- Pam Niederer, R.N., Clinical Services Manager, Surgical Center of York, York, PA

- Alexandra Reyes, R.N., Administrator, Treasure Coast Center for Surgery, Stuart, FL

- Darlene Mashman, M.D., Assistant Professor of Anesthesiology, Emory University School of Medicine, Atlanta

We are grateful to The Joint Commission staff reviewed this book: Michael Kulczycki, Lon Berkeley, Beverly Robins, Virginia McCollum, Joyce Webb, Deborah Nadzam, Michael Jarema, and Diane Bell. And special thanks to writer Andrea M. Sattinger for her efforts in crafting this book.

References

1. Kohn L.T., Corrigan J.M., Donaldson M.S.: Institute of Medicine Committee on Quality of Health Care in America. *To Err Is Human: Building a Safer Health System.* Washington, DC: National Academy Press, 1999.
2. Plews-Ogan M.L., et al.: Patient safety in the ambulatory setting. A clinician-based approach. *J Gen Intern Med* 19:719–725, Jul. 2004.
3. O'Reilly K.B.: Spotlight shifts to outpatient safety. *Am Med News* 49:14, Jun. 12, 2006.
4. Woods D.M, et al.: Ambulatory care adverse events and preventable adverse events leading to a hospital admission. *Qual Saf Health Care* 16:127–131, Apr. 2007.
5. Elder N.C., Pallerla H., Regan S.: What do family physicians consider an error? A comparison of definitions and physician perception. *BMC Fam Pract* 7:73, Dec. 8, 2006.
6. Sabogal F., Snow A., Sawyer L.: The business case for patient safety. *CAHQ Journal* 32:10–16, 27–34, Jan.–Mar. 2008.
7. Reason J.: Understanding adverse events: The human factor. In London V.C. (ed.): *Clinical Risk Management: Enhancing Patient Safety.* London: BMJ Publications, 2001.
8. The Joint Commission: *Cost-Effective Performance Improvement in Ambulatory Care.* Oakbrook Terrace, IL: Joint Commission Resources, 2002.
9. The Joint Commission: *Sentinel Event.* 2009. http://www.jointcommission.org/SentinelEvents/ (accessed May 7, 2009).
10. Heckinger E., et al.: Disease management: A mid-decade evolution toward patient safety. *Home Health Care Management & Practice* 18:178–185, Apr. 2006.
11. Runy L.A.: Outpatient services and ED visits continue to climb. *Hosp Health Netw* 80:36, Mar. 2006.
12. Kairys J.A.: Top 5 causes of medical errors in ambulatory care. *For*

the Business of Medicine, PRI-MED Patient Education Center, Jan. 2007. http://www.patientedu.org/aspx/News/news_detail.aspx?newsid=219 (accessed Feb. 6, 2009).

13. Gandhi T.K., et al.: Missed and delayed diagnoses in the ambulatory setting: A study of closed malpractice claims. *Ann Intern Med* 145:488–496, Oct. 3, 2006.

14. Singh R., et al.: Prioritizing threats to patient safety in rural primary care. *J Rural Health* 23:173–178, Spring 2007.

15. Wachter R.W.: *Is Ambulatory Patient Safety Just Like Hospital Safety, Only Without the "Stat"?* PowerPoint presentation. Michigan Health and Safety Coalition Annual Patient Safety Conference, Troy, MI, Mar. 28–29, 2007. http://www.mihealthandsafety.org/patientsafety2007/9.pdf (accessed Mar. 8, 2009).

16. The Joint Commission: *Engaging Physicians in Patient Safety: A Handbook for Leaders.* Oakbrook Terrace, IL: Joint Commission Resources, 2006.

17. The Joint Commission: Preventing pediatric medication errors. *Sentinel Event Alert* 39, Apr. 11, 2008. http://www.jointcommission.org/SentinelEvents/SentinelEventAlert/sea_39.htm (accessed May 12, 2009).

Chapter 1

PATIENT-CENTERED CARE

The term *patient-centered medicine* was introduced by Balint and colleagues in 1969.[1] In 1988, the term *patient-centered care* was coined by the Picker Commonwealth Program for Patient-Centered Care, which then became the Picker Institute. As described by Planetree, a nonprofit collaborative education and information organization, patient-centered care is the core of a high-quality health care system and a necessary foundation for safe, effective, efficient, timely, and equitable care.[2] Planetree's model of patient-centered care expresses the essential theme that health care should be delivered in a manner that works best for patients.[2]

The Institute of Medicine's 2001 seminal report, *Crossing the Quality Chasm,* identified patient-centeredness as an essential foundation for quality and patient safety.[3] The report went against the grain of the conventional perspective of a patient-centered approach. Patient-centered care was more than just a peripheral aim. This effectively ushered in a reorientation of the U.S. health care delivery system as one in which the way care is delivered is considered equally as important as the care itself.[4,5]

As it relates to patient safety, organizations practicing patient-centered care recognize that each patient is a unique person and has diverse needs. Given that, patients must be considered as partners; consulting with them to gain their special knowledge about themselves can reduce risks of adverse events. In addition, patients' family and friends are also partners who can help to maintain safety when the patient is undergoing care in the ambulatory setting. Empowering patients to participate in their care is a fundamental component of safe care.

For example, patient-centered care underlies the concept of medical home initiatives, which serve as models of personalized care coordination to deliver access and care for chronic disease beyond treatment for acute-care episodes.[6,7]

Patient-centered care involves serving the individual patient in terms of his or her language, culture, ethnicity, preferences, medical and psychosocial history, and contextual issues (particular issues in his or her life and lifestyle, and those of his or her family or other caregivers, which may adversely affect adherence to treatment recommendations). A patient safety program provides a strong base for good communication. An excellent tool for use with overall patient safety assessment is presented in Figure 1-1, page 2.

Issues of safety that relate to patient-centric and family-centric care include errors in diagnosis, the use of information technology, truly informed consent, patient and family safety reports, patient identification, and patient education.

Delayed or Missed Diagnoses

Delays in making a correct diagnosis may result in patients receiving the wrong treatment or in a potentially serious condition becoming worse. Patients often present to ambulatory organizations with multiple symptoms, concerns, and complaints. The right diagnosis and treatment regimen are needed to reduce symptoms and help patients meet their health objectives.

Any dialogue between patient and provider is educational, including the history taking. Other issues that call for concerted communication and education of patients to maintain safety include medication reconciliation activities (informing them of current medications, and so on), communicating test results or directing patients to have tests done, or explaining to patients about referrals to other providers. The patient

Figure 1-1. Sample Outline for a Patient Safety Plan

Program goals (consistent with organization mission)

Scope of the program
- Activities & functions relating to patient safety (*TIP: Dig deeper for ideas on program components.*)
- Participating sites, settings, and services

Structure
- Management of the program (*TIP: Regardless of the size of the practice, be sure to designate a patient safety officer.*)
- Components (safety-related offices, committees, functions)
- Interdisciplinary participation (*TIP: In larger practices, include representatives of all clinical and administrative disciplines in the practice. For smaller practices, include everyone. In all cases, include every member of the staff in various patient safety activities. Remember: Safety is a team sport!*)
- Oversight

Mechanisms for coordination
- Among components of the program
- Among the professional disciplines
- Across the organization

Communicating with patients about safety
- Patient education
- Informing patients about their care

Staff education
- Safety-related orientation & training (*TIP: Establish a training agenda each year and stick to it; update topic areas based on patient safety leaders' monthly newsletters and other sources of patient safety news and innovations.*)
- Team training
- Expectations for reporting (*TIP: Establish monthly tracking of key patient safety statistics and post in a public space.*)

Safety improvement activities
- Definition of terms
- Prioritization of improvement activities
- Routine safety-related data collection and analysis
  —Incident reporting
  —Medication error reporting
  —Infection surveillance
  —Facility safety surveillance
  —Staff perceptions of and suggestions for improving patient safety
  —Staff willingness to report errors
  —Patient/family perceptions of and suggestions for improving patient safety
- Identification, reporting, and management of sentinel events
- Proactive risk reduction
  –Identification of high-risk processes
  –Failure mode, effects, and criticality analysis
- Reporting of results
  –To the patient safety program
  –To organization staff
  –To executive leadership and the governing body

This sample outline can serve as the foundation for building effective communication strategies. Access this and other tools online at http://www.pathwaysforpatientsafety.org.

Source: Pathways for Patient Safety. Health Research and Educational Trust, Institute for Safe Medication Practices, Medical Group Management Association, 2008.

truly is the one "health care team member" who stays the same in any health setting he or she goes to. In many ways, staff (including nonclinical staff) can encourage patients to recognize and share critical information with their health care providers.

Errors in diagnosis may be linked to poor history taking or communication breakdowns. Experts at Kaiser Permanente found that in the adverse events involving some of their 8.4 million members, 44% of demands for payment and liability lawsuits arose from missed or delayed diagnoses. Of these[8]:

- 55% were failures to order appropriate diagnostic or laboratory tests (*see* Chapter 2).
- 44% had inappropriate or inadequate follow-up.
- 38% were incorrect interpretation of diagnostic or laboratory tests (*see* Chapter 2).
- 31% came from an inadequately performed physical exam.

A study conducted by ProMutual Group insurance found that in primary care and radiology, errors in diagnosis were the leading allegations in more than half of lawsuits.[9] The research also found that undetected cancer was involved in 47% of failure-to-diagnose claims. Most of the misdiagnosis claims were traced back to lack of patient history and a lack of follow-up.

Although most health care organizations view diagnosis error as a clinical failure, research suggests that these errors are often related to faulty systems in an organization. The system-level elements usually found in these cases include cultural acceptance of suboptimal systems, inadequate policies and procedures, inefficient processes, and problems with teamwork and communication.[10]

Solutions for improving the visibility of diagnostic errors include the following[10,11–15]:

- Include diagnostic error in the normal spectrum of quality assurance surveillance and review.
- Create simple definitions and rules to identify, classify, and study errors.
- Differentiate the origins of errors regarding whether any elements are provider specific (pertain to cognitive errors), system related, or "no fault" (that is, reflecting diseases and conditions with atypical presentations or that involve excessive patient nonadherence to treatment plans).

- Consider and implement ways to provide feedback to clinicians regarding their diagnoses.
- Identify how communication processes may result in faulty or absent information, leading to diagnostic errors.
- Implement reliable processes for diagnostic testing, and, as mentioned above, address timeliness in communicating abnormal test results.
- Consider requiring mandatory second opinions and computer-assisted decision support in the perceptual specialties—pathology and radiology—and clinical decision support tools in other settings where surveillance reveals excessive errors.
- Encourage clinicians to learn about diagnostic errors and reflect on their own level of overconfidence about cognitive thinking deficits.

Diagnostic error: A diagnosis that is missed, wrong, or delayed, as detected by some subsequent test or finding.[10]

Information Technology

Having all the information you need when you need it is important to safety and quality in all health care settings. How can providers in different ambulatory settings communicate in real time about patient treatment needs when their systems are not integrated within one system? Information technology (IT) innovations can balance communication needs and access to clinical information needed to make patient-centered decisions.

The quality and level of an organization's IT may affect a patient's care in positive or negative ways. Examples of IT include Internet, electronic mail, electronic medical records (electronic health records), computerized prescriber order entry, and clinical decision support systems. In a study of voluntary reporting of adverse events and near misses in a large internal medicine practice, 47% of the reported errors involved medications.[16] Of the 70 interventions recommended by the physician research team, more than half were potentially preventable by an electronic prescribing system with decision support keyed to patients' electronic medical records.

Tips for incorporating IT in the ambulatory setting include the following:

- Designate a multidisciplinary electronic medical

records team to meet regularly to discuss system-related issues.

- Plan staff educational programs.
- Share updates on any system modifications.
- Consider and budget for purchases.

Electronic medical records, sometimes called electronic health records, hold a number of benefits in ambulatory health care (AHC). Unfortunately, at this time, fewer than 25% of ambulatory providers have instituted electronic medical records. Rural areas and underserved communities may represent the most challenging environments to implement expensive technological solutions. However, IT may represent a potential solution to disparities in care because decision support is delivered for all patients, access to up-to-date health information is improved, long-distance clinical consultation or delivery of health care through telemedicine can be facilitated, and more effective population management is possible.

Many clinical settings are trying to implement IT systems for computerized prescriber order entry, orders, and medication reconciliation and verification. But implementing IT for health care can be much harder than it looks, and when installed, systems may not remedy problems as expected. The Joint Commission suggests several actions for avoiding problems associated with implementing health care IT.[17] Many low-tech solutions can also be used to keep patients safe (*see also* "Filing System Errors," page 14 in Chapter 2).

TOOL: IT Solutions

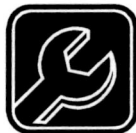

The functions available in electronic health records (as well as the extent to which physicians use them) vary considerably.[18] For example, computerized drug prescribing alerts can improve patient safety, but alerts are often overridden because of poor specificity and alert overload. A study conducted at 31 ambulatory care practices in the Boston area is relevant for other ambulatory practices. The study aimed to improve clinician acceptance of drug alerts. A selective set of drug alerts for the ambulatory care setting was designed, allowing minimal workflow disruptions by designating only critical to high-severity alerts to be interruptive to clinician workflow.[19] The authors learned that a balance must be reached to avoid over-alerting. By implementing tiered alerts, they limited alert burden by assigning 71% of triggered alerts to a noninterruptive display mode. By interrupting clinicians for only those drug contraindications with the highest clinical importance, they could achieve fewer interruptive alerts and greater clinician acceptance of alerts.[19]

Truly Informed Consent

One paramount safety (and quality) responsibility of health care providers is giving patients the necessary information to make informed decisions. When patients sign an informed consent sheet, this does not ensure that they understand the process or the risks they are about to face. The pages are long, the language is sometimes formidable, and the timing is often poor. The patient has already agreed to undergo the procedure, and the paperwork seems just an obligatory routine. That is not the way to provide safe care. The patient needs to know up front the risks and benefits *and* understand them (*see also* "Patient Education," beginning on page 7 in this chapter, and Chapter 7, "Staff Education and Training," beginning on page 105).

The Speak Up™ program of The Joint Commission is an excellent way to better equip patients to think and act on behalf of their own care. Educate and encourage your patients to speak up and to ask as many questions as they need to. A number of Speak Up brochures are available from The Joint Commission Web site.

Patient and Family Safety Reports

Joint Commission requirements call for identifying ways in which patients and families can report concerns about safety, and taking the time to encourage them to do so.

Health care safety experts agree that changing the culture of safety is paramount in reducing rates of medical errors. Part of the necessary culture change is to encourage and welcome the involvement of patients and their families in reporting adverse events or potential safety issues. The lack of effective communication between patients and providers contributes to safety risks. Receptivity to reports from patients is fundamental to preventing risks. Encouraging patients and families to participate in error-reduction efforts includes supporting patient education (*see* pages 7–11 in this chapter).

As explained in an article published by the Agency for Healthcare Research and Quality (AHRQ), patients have three roles in improving patient safety, and organizations should make them aware of these roles.[20] Patients can do the following:

- Help ensure their own safety
- Work with their providers and health care practices to improve safety at the organization and unit level
- Advocate as citizens for public reporting and accountability of health system performance

Physician practices as well as other ambulatory settings should include a means of reporting errors and potentials risks for harm in their policies and procedures. Do not leave this up to the paperwork, however. Encourage staff to emphasize that patients are not only welcome to question procedures and actions, but that they should speak up.

TOOL: Reprisal-Free Error Reporting

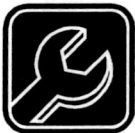

Error rates will never be reduced if people do not feel comfortable reporting errors. The organization must work over time to establish a just culture wherein practitioners and other staff report and openly discuss errors without undo embarrassment or fear of reprisal from management. A just culture balances the response of the health care system to error between holding the error maker completely responsible and holding the system completely to blame. As it strikes a balance between a punitive environment and a "blame-free" culture, such a culture differentiates between individual behaviors and system failures. It recognizes that humans do make errors and should be held accountable for risky and reckless behaviors.

A tool designed by Creighton University for ambulatory care is presented in Figure 1-2, pages 6–7.

Patient Identification

Every organization should establish a well-publicized process for patient identification. Verify information by asking the patient, or the family, the patient's date of birth and name. Compare this information against your order or requisition. Periodically survey these practices to maintain compliance with the organization's patient identification policy.

✓ Joint Commission requirements call for at least two patient identifiers when providing treatment and services.

Procedures performed in ambulatory surgery centers may require patient identification practices that are just as intricate as those performed in inpatient surgical suites. Procedures performed in the AHC surgical setting require advance scheduling, including the name of the patient, medical record number, name of the procedure, surgeon's name and contact information, type of anesthesia, length of procedure, special equipment, pathology requests, blood and blood products, and other general information. Collecting this information allows staff to obtain the correct instruments and equipment, blood and blood products, and appropriate complement of nursing and surgical technicians, as well as any special requests for radiologic procedures and pathology services during the procedure. Communication deficits that lead to canceling procedures (for instance, for lack of specialty supplies) may result in delayed diagnosis if the facility must cancel a diagnostic procedure. Patient identification is necessary, therefore, not only to ensure that the proper patient is receiving the proper treatment, but also to enable staff to proactively prepare for the patient's (and providers') needs.

✓ The Joint Commission calls for preventing transfusion errors with the use of careful patient identification.

Transfusion Safety

In some AHC organizations, patient misidentification creates an issue with transfusion safety, which is distinctly different from blood component safety. Although blood safety focuses on ensuring a low risk of disease transmission in prepared blood products, transfusion safety is concerned with the entire process of delivering the component to the patient. Infectious risks of transfusion have been dramatically reduced, but the noninfectious risks have received relatively less attention.[21]

Figure 1-2. Error Management in a Just Culture

Medication Safety Best Practices Guide

ERROR MANAGEMENT	Level	Satisfactory
When medication errors or adverse reactions come to the attention of the clinic staff, the following takes place: • staff involved with the error or adverse reaction review the circumstances involved. • entire staff are provided with service education and training. • policies and procedures are reviewed and revised if necessary to prevent a reoccurrence.	2	
Prescribers and clinic staff involved in serious errors that caused a patient harm are offered psychological counseling as well as emotional support by their colleagues.	2	
Staff who are directly involved in a serious or potentially seerous medication error participate in analyzing those failures in the system that allowed the error to happen and are encouraged to recommend system enhancements to reduce the potential for errors.	2	
As a matter of practice, medication errors and ways to avoid them are openly discussed between prescribers and clinic staff.	1	
Individuals are not dismissed from employment because of a medication error in this office.[19]	2	
Prescribers and nurses receive ongoing information regarding medication errors occurring within the organization, error-prone situations, errors occurring in other clinics, and strategies to prevent such errors.[19]	2	
Ongoing information regarding medication errors is communicated to staff members: • verbally at the time of the medication error. • by written communication. • at regularly scheduled clinical staff meetings.	2	
Reference to errors is not included in employee personnel files.[19]	2	
Errors are not considered as a performance measure during either annual performance appraisals or during competency assessments.[19,20]	2	
Management provides positive incentives for individuals to report errors.[21]	2	
Prescribers and clinic staff are reacted to in a positive manner for detecting and reporting errors.	2	
There is an integrated plan to detect, analyze and reduce medication errors in the clinic with at least one staff member responsible for the plan.[19]	2	

CHRP   Kimberly A. Galt Pharm. D. and Ann M. Rule Pharm. D. © 2004 Creighton University Health Services Research Program

(continued on page 7)

The transfusion of blood to the wrong patient—that is, mistransfusion—is the most serious safety risk, occurring in 1 in 19,000 transfusions.[21] The risks include a fatal hemolytic transfusion reaction, transfusing ABO-incompatible blood, and transfusions of viral and other microbiologic products.

AHC–specific solutions for patient identification to avoid a mistransfusion include[22]:
■ A well-organized blood program, which guarantees a safe, adequate, and timely supply
■ The availability of simple alternatives for transfusion (crystalloids and colloids) for the correction of hypo-

Figure 1-2. Error Management in a Just Culture (continued)

ERROR MANAGEMENT	Level	Satisfactory
The patient care process is specifically evaluated for opportunities to reduce errors at least annually. [19]	2	
Clear definitions and examples of medication errors and hazardous situations that should be reported have been established for use in this clinic.	2	
A formal system is in place for reporting hazardous situations that could lead to an error. [22]	2	
A formal system is in place for reporting actual errors.	2	
"Near misses" that have potential to cause harm are given the same high priority for analysis and error prevention strategies as errors that actually cause patient harm. [20]	2	
Prescribers use published error experiences from their organization to proactively target improvement in the prescribing process.	1	
Prescribers report to external voluntary reporting programs such as the USP Medication Errors Reporting Program, FDA MedWatch or the CDC Vaccine Adverse Reaction Reporting Program.	1	
If the prescriber discovers that an error has led to improper medication prescribing regardless of the level of harm that results, the error is disclosed to the patient/caregiver/family.	1	

This tool can reduce staff anxiety about reprisal from reporting mishaps and errors. Implementation levels: 1 = Implementation requires no additional resources. The solution is accomplished through changes in individual behavior to achieve safety improvement. 2 = Implementation requires no additional resources. The solution is accomplished through change in policy or system(s). A third level, not indicated in this example, calls for solutions accomplished through additional financial or expert resources beyond those currently available in ambulatory care.

Source: Creighton Health Services Research Program (CHRP), Creighton University: *Medication Safety Best Practices Guide for Ambulatory Care Use.* http://chrp.creighton.edu/documents/bestpractices.pdf (accessed May 12, 2009). Permission given as open access.

volemia, and pharmaceuticals and medical devices to reduce blood loss
■ The education and training of clinicians, nurses, and blood transfusion service staff involved in the transfusion process

Patient Education

Joint Commission requirements call for encouraging patients' active involvement in their own care, and this serves doubly as a patient safety strategy. Involving patients and families means helping educate them about what they should expect for their care and the importance of their roles in reporting perceived risks to their care. To describe and explain these patient responsibilities, organizations should educate individuals about the following, verbally, in writing, or both[23]:
■ The plan for care, treatment, and services
■ Basic health practices and safety
■ The safe and effective use of medications
■ Nutrition interventions, modified diets, or oral health
■ Safe and effective use of medical equipment or supplies when provided by the organization
■ Understanding pain, the risk for pain, the importance of effective pain management, the pain assessment process, and methods for pain management
■ Habilitation or rehabilitation techniques to help them

reach the maximum independence possible
- Infection control, hand hygiene, personal protection precautions

Reducing errors and improving the safety of care requires the coordinated efforts of many individuals, not the least of which are patients themselves.[24] Patients can help identify potential errors as they observe and participate in the care process. But patients may not always bring up problems or ask questions about issues that concern them. The first step, therefore, is to empower patients to participate in their own care by emphasizing the importance of their participation. Encourage patients to bring up any questions or concerns. Involving patients in care first means involving yourself in their concerns and interests. A template for involving patients in their own care is presented in Table 1-1 on this page.

Effective patient education involves giving patients what they need in order to receive the right information at the right time in the right manner. Issues that must be taken into account when effecting this goal include diversity, literacy, and the ways in which communication takes place.

Cultural and diversity issues among patients impact their health care, as has been demonstrated in abundant research over several decades.[25] Implement a policy to individualize care for patients with particular diversity issues such as ethnicity, language, cultural values, religious practices and health beliefs, gender, age, education, and sexual orientation, including transgender.

One excellent example of incorporating a "best practice" that respects the need to accommodate staff diversity as well as diversity in educating patients was incorporated by the Bureau of Prisons Federal Correctional Complex facilities in Tucson, Arizona. The AHC facility there prominently posted the National Patient Safety Goals in both English and Spanish in exam rooms. More than 40% of the facility speaks Spanish, and the facility also has many bilingual staff and inmates.

Low literacy is a pervasive problem in health care. Approximately 21% of American adults are functionally illiterate, and another 27% have marginal literacy skills.[26] Such patients may have difficulty reading and

Table 1-1. How to Involve Patients in Their Own Care
1. Converse and communicate. Make sure the patient understands what you are saying and make sure you understand what the patient is saying.
2. Listen. Repeat back your understanding of what you heard.
3. Invite, encourage, and welcome patients to take more responsibility and involvement with their own care. This does not take long and won't interfere with your work and schedule. It takes only a matter of seconds to communicate sincerely, genuinely, and compassionately. Most patients will engage more in their care when they perceive their providers to be partners.
4. Some patients are extremely reluctant to become involved in their own care. They may want you and others (family, friends) to be the informed decision makers. It may be a challenge to involve such patients. Family may help. Someone on the staff may also have more connection or facility with a particular patient.
5. Recommend approved Web sites. Many patients use online sources for health and health care information. Supply Web site addresses in writing and tell patients which ones they can trust.
6. Supply written instructions and educational materials.
7. Be personable. Suggestions from any health care provider can go a long way toward supporting a patient in becoming healthier and health conscious.
8. Support patients in completing and filing advance directives.
9. Be receptive to patients' interests in medicine other than conventional medicine. You turn off a patient if you dismiss his or her thoughts, questions, and beliefs.
10. Treat patients with respect. Always.
11. Encourage good health and healthy lifestyles as opposed to only responding to illness.

understanding discharge instructions, medication labels, patient education materials, consent forms, or health surveys. In the ambulatory setting, low literacy particularly contributes to medical and medication non-adherence. Lower literacy and taking a greater number of medications have been associated with patient misunderstanding of pill bottle labels.[27] Properly assessing the literacy level of individual patients, or groups of patients, may help avoid problems in clinical care.

Researchers at two hospital-based primary care clinics and one federally qualified health center in Chicago, New York, and Shreveport, Louisiana, tested whether using more explicit language to describe dose and frequency of use for prescribed drugs could improve comprehension, particularly among patients with limited literacy.[27] With 359 adults waiting for an appointment in one of the ambulatory sites, surveys collected data on correct understanding of each of 10 label instructions as determined by a blinded panel review of patients' verbatim responses. Patient understanding of prescription label instructions ranged from 53% for the least understood to 89% for the most commonly understood label. Patients were significantly more likely to understand dosage instructions with explicit time periods (that is, morning) or precise times of day compared to instructions stating a number of times per day (that is, twice) or hourly intervals. Low and marginal literacy remained statistically significant independent predictors of misinterpreting instructions.

Problems associated with literacy include more than whether a patient can read and write. It is also important for staff to consider the way they themselves are talking, including the buzz words or jargon they may use when communicating with patients and families. An effective and quick tool to use to assess a patient's reading level is the REALM literacy test, the most commonly used test of health literacy, which assesses a patient's word recognition of 66 terms. The REALM literacy test, as well as other useful tools, links, and patient education brochures, is available at the Indian Health Service Health Education Program Web site, which is listed along with other online resources in Sidebar 1-1, right.

Patient Involvement and Responsibility

Helping patients assume more responsibility for their care means moving beyond the following assumptions:

- They can read and understand the provider's intentions and instructions.
- Their culture accepts what is detailed in the provided care plans.
- They have no role to play in adhering to treatment and their own wellness.

A number of tools and techniques can be used so patients will better handle their medications and other

---

Sidebar 1-1. Online Resources for Patient and Family Education

For patients and other consumers:

Indian Health Service Health Education Program
http://www.ihs.gov/NonMedicalPrograms/HealthEd/index.cfm

Consumers Advancing Patient Safety (CAPS)
http://www.patientsafety.org/

National Patient Safety Foundation
http://www.npsf.org

National Agenda for Action: Patients and Families in Patient Safety
http://www.npsf.org/pdf/paf/AgendaFamilies.pdf

Informed Medical Decisions
http://www.informedmedicaldecisions.org/

Resources for professionals that include patient education materials:

AHRQ Patient Safety Network
http://psnet.ahrq.gov

AHRQ *WebM&M*
http://www.webmm.ahrq.gov

AHRQ Advances in Patient Safety: From Research to Implementation
http://www.ahrq.gov/qual/advances

U.S. Department of Veterans Affairs (VA) National Center for Patient Safety
http://www.va.gov/ncps/index.html

National Patient Safety Foundation
http://www.npsf.org

---

aspects of safety[28]:

- Purchase or create pamphlets on the topic of safe use of medications.
- Discuss the importance of checking meds often and reporting any side effects to their providers.
- Provide patients with copies of their medication list.
- Consider using a convenient tool for patients such as a "health passport" in English and other languages.
- Urge patients to regularly bring in their medications for a checkup.
- Encourage elderly and chronically ill patients to assess their risk level for home safety: fire, falls, and medications.
- Consider developing a Patient Safety Advisory Council on topics of interest and importance to patients and their families.

Sidebar 1-2. Communicating with Patients to Prevent and Reduce Errors

The Dana-Farber Cancer Institute in Boston examined the potential value of a patient-oriented teamwork intervention by developing and conducting a teamwork-training initiative for oncology patients and their families. The content and format of the initiative, conducted from July through September 2007, was based on several core team-training concepts derived from the research literature in health care and aviation. The You CAN campaign sought to convey a positive and empowering message that encouraged patients to (1) check for hazards in the environment, (2) ask questions of clinicians, and (3) notify staff of safety concerns.

Based on safety principles such as situational awareness and closed-loop communication, the intervention focused on encouraging patients to ask specific questions regarding their care. Thirty-two percent of the ambulatory clinic population, or 1,145 patients, were exposed to the campaign, and 39% of those who were exposed to the campaign said that the intervention changed their behavior to be more involved in their care.

You CAN Campaign Messages for Patients were to do the following:
- **Check.** To convey the concept of *situational awareness*, the campaign encouraged patients to pay attention to the details of their care and to check at each visit to make sure things "looked right."
    - Was their chemotherapy the same color as it was at the last treatment?
    - Were their pills the same color and shape?
    - Recognizing that sick patients may not feel capable of this kind of vigilance, patients were encouraged to bring along a friend or family member, when possible, as an extra set of eyes and ears.

- **Ask.** Asking questions was a way for patients to actively engage with their caregivers by employing *appropriate assertiveness*. Patients were encouraged to do the following:
    - Ask about the potential side effects of their medicines and how best to manage them
    - Ask their health care providers if they washed their hands and to repeat anything the patients did not hear or understand. By asking for clarification and repeating important information aloud, patients could utilize *closed-loop communication* to ensure that messages were acknowledged and understood.

- **Notify.** To facilitate the exchange of new information among patients and providers, the campaign urged patients to *brief* their caregivers about any side effects they had experienced between visits and any significant changes to their care. Specifically, patients could relay any last-minute changes physicians had made to treatment orders to the nurses at infusion, minimizing the possibility of chemotherapy misadministration.

Source: Weingart S.N., et al.: The You CAN campaign: Teamwork training for patients and families in ambulatory oncology. *Jt Comm J Qual Patient Saf* 35:63–71, Feb. 2009.

- Consider supplying pill boxes for patients on multiple medications.

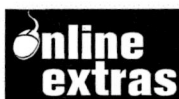

Online extras The Spanish and English versions of the patient medication document used at Baptist Health South Florida are available on our Web site: http://www.jcrinc.com/PSAC09/extras/.

Regardless of the AHC setting, the amount of time providers have with patients is generally minimal. Careful communication is extremely important to ensure quality and eliminate risks to safety. Sidebar 1-2, above, presents tips suggested by the You CAN campaign for communicating with patients to prevent errors.

TOOL: Telephone-Based Disease Management Support Program

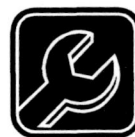

Interactive telephone technology can be used as a tool to support a disease management program. A collaborative team of researchers from the Division of General Internal Medicine at the University of California–San Francisco used an automated telephone self-management support program for diabetes patients as an opportunity to monitor patient safety.[29]

The project identified adverse and potential adverse events among a diverse group of diabetes patients participating in an automated telephone health IT self-

---

Table 1-2. Adopting the Telephone-Based Diabetes Management Program

Getting Started with This Initiative

The following are needed to implement this program effectively:

- Leadership buy-in to support the cost and effort involved
- One or more clinical champions
- Capacity for interactive voice response or automated calling
- Automated phone scripts (which can be developed or purchased)
- A trained nurse or response team
- A diabetes registry or list of persons eligible for and/or in need of ongoing monitoring

Sustaining This Initiative

- Seek ways to reduce per-patient costs. For example, multiple clinics could collaborate on the project or could implement it in conjunction with a payer health plan.

Other Considerations

- Consider linking this program to a strategy designed to increase medication compliance, which has greater potential for a positive impact on metabolic measures (for example, blood glucose, lipid levels)

Source: University of California–San Francisco, Division of General Internal Medicine.

---

management program via weekly interactions augmented by targeted nurse follow-up. Among the 111 patients, they identified 111 adverse events and 153 potential adverse events. Of completed calls, 11% detected an event. Close to 60% of events were detected through health IT–facilitated triggers, followed by nurse elicitation (30%), and patient callback requests (11%). The majority of events (93%) were categorized as preventable or ameliorable. Primary care providers were aware of only 13% of incidents (one-time) and 60% of prevalent (pervasive) events.[29] A short summary of some considerations in adopting this initiative is presented in Table 1-2, above.

References

1. Balint M., Ball D.H., Hare M.L.: Training medical students in patient-centered medicine. *Compr Psychiatry* 10:249–258, Jul. 1969.
2. Frampton S., et al.: *Patient-Centered Care Improvement Guide.* Planetree and Picker Institute. Oct. 2008. http://www.ihi.org/IHI/Topics/PatientCenteredCare/ (accessed May 12, 2009).
3. Institute of Medicine: *Crossing the Quality Chasm: A New Health System for the 21st Century.* Washington, DC: National Academy Press, 2001.
4. Berwick D.M.: A user's manual for the IOM's "Quality Chasm" report. *Health Aff* 21:80–90, May–Jun. 2002.
5. Battles J.B.: Quality and safety by design. *Qual Saf Health Care* 15(suppl. 1):i1–i3, 2006.
6. American Academy of Family Physicians, American Academy of Pediatrics, American College of Physicians, American Osteopathic Association: *Joint Principles of the Patient-Centered Medical Home.* Mar. 2007. http://www.medicalhomeinfo.org/ (accessed May 11, 2009).
7. Baron R.J.: The chasm between intention and achievement in primary care. *JAMA* 301:1922–1924, May 13, 2009.
8. O'Reilly K.B.: Spotlight shifts to outpatient safety. *Am Med News.* 49:14, Jun. 12, 2006.
9. Sorrel A.L.: Failure to diagnose is the No. 1 allegation in liability lawsuits. *Am Med News* 49:13, 15, Mar. 20, 2006.
10. Graber M.: Diagnostic errors in medicine: A case of neglect. In Schiff G.D. (ed.): *Getting Results: Reliably Communicating and Acting on Critical Test Results.* Oakbrook Terrace, IL: Joint Commission Resources, 2006, pp. 125–133.
11. Graber M.L., Franklin N., Gordon R.: Diagnostic error in internal medicine. *Arch Intern Med* 165:1493–1499, Jul. 11, 2005.
12. Groopman J.: *How Doctors Think.* New York: Houghton Mifflin Company, 2007.
13. Schiff G.D., et al.: *Diagnosing Diagnosis Errors: Lessons from a Multi-Institutional Collaborative Project.* Rockville, MD: Agency for Healthcare Research and Quality (Publication No. 050021-2.), 2005.
14. Weiner S.J., et al.: Evaluating physician performance at individualizing care: A pilot study tracking contextual errors in medical decision making. *Med Decis Making* 27:726–734, Nov.–Dec. 2007.
15. Trowbridge R.L.: Twelve tips for teaching avoidance of diagnostic errors. *Med Teach* 30:496–500, Jun. 2008.
16. Plews-Ogan M.L., et al.: Patient safety in the ambulatory setting. A clinician-based approach. *J Gen Intern Med* 19:719–725, Jul. 2004.
17. Mitka M.: Joint Commission offers warnings, advice on adopting new health care IT Systems. *JAMA* 301:587–589, Feb. 11, 2009.
18. Simon S.R., et al.: Physicians and electronic health records: A statewide survey. *Arch Intern Med* 167:507–512, Mar. 12, 2007.
19. Shah N.R., et al.: Improving acceptance of computerized prescribing alerts in ambulatory care. *J Am Med Inform Assoc* 13:5–11, Jan.–Feb. 2006.
20. Gibson R.: The role of the patient in improving patient safety. *Web M&M,* Agency for Healthcare Research and Quality. http://www.webmm.ahrq.gov/perspective.aspx? perspectiveID=38 (accessed Mar. 3, 2009).
21. Brown M.R., Fitsma M.G., Marques M.B.: Transfusion safety: What has been done; what is still needed? *MLO Med Lab Obs* 37:20,22–23,26, Nov. 2005.
22. World Health Organization: *Blood Transfusion Safety. Safe and Appropriate Use.* http://www.who.int/bloodsafety/clinical_use/en/ (accessed Mar. 8, 2009).
23. Greiner A.C., Knebel E. (eds.): *Health Professions Education: A Bridge to Quality.* Washington, DC: Institute of Medicine, 2003.
24. The Joint Commission: *Engaging Physicians in Patient Safety: A Handbook for Leaders.* Oakbrook Terrace, IL: Joint Commission Resources, 2006.
25. Department of Health and Human Services, National Institutes of Health, Centers for Disease Control and Prevention, National

Institute for Occupational Safety and Health: *Research Supplements to Promote Diversity in Health-Related Research.* http://grants.nih.gov/grants/guide/pa-files/PA-08-190.html (accessed May 10, 2009).

26. Davis T.C., et al.: Practical assessment of adult literacy in health care. *Health Educ Behav* 25:613–624, Oct. 1998.

27. Davis T.C., et al.: Improving patient understanding of prescription drug label instructions. *J Gen Intern Med* 24:57–62, Jan. 2009.

28. Schauberger C., et al.: *Ambulatory Patient Safety Toolkit. Safety Collaborative for the OutPatient Environment (SCOPE). Gundersen Lutheran Health System.* Oct. 2003. http://www.gundluth.org/ (accessed Feb. 9, 2009).

29. Sarkar U., et al.: Use of an interactive, telephone-based self-management support program to identify adverse events among ambulatory diabetes patients. *J Gen Intern Med* 23, Aug. 29, 2008. http://www.innovations.ahrq.gov/ content.aspx?id=1863 (accessed May 14, 2009).

Chapter 2
COMMUNICATION

Effective communication is essential for optimal patient outcomes, and poor communication can lead to patient harm and injury. Communication issues associated with patient safety are composed of two main categories: preventing adverse events and responding to adverse events.

The Joint Commission has consistently reported that communication problems are at the core of most of the sentinel event reports it receives. An episode of ambulatory care may require coordination and communication among many individuals at many sites, including clinicians, the patient and family, external laboratories, and imaging facilities.

Communication breakdowns can occur in various ways: at patient handoffs (for example, at patient discharge from the hospital when responsibility for care is now transferred back to the primary care provider), within the team of caregivers in a particular setting (such as in surgery or a dialysis unit), between two providers or organizations (such as with the processing of test results), and between a provider and a patient or the patient's family.

Joint Commission requirements call for improving the effectiveness of communication among caregivers[1] and encouraging patients' active involvement in their own care as a patient safety strategy. Both are highly dependent on conducting effective communication.

A number of important issues are associated with ineffective communication in health care, including filing system errors, telephone and verbal orders, and problems during transitions of care (handoffs). The appropriate use of electronic communication tools is also essential. Specific high-risk communication areas include medication management, laboratory testing, and imaging. This chapter will review the general points for effective communication and how to improve communication in those specific areas.

Improving Communication

Communication is a two-way street. The dynamics between a patient and provider will impact care. Human factors affect the relationship, which in turn can affect the outcome. Bring into the mix the influence of other providers, poorly designed or lack of effective processes of care, and/or breakdowns in those processes, and you have a formula for potential lapses in safety.

A study from a decade ago concerning medical encounters in ambulatory health care (AHC) concluded that clinicians perceive one in six patient encounters as being difficult.[2] Such perception affects exchange of information and can adversely affect outcomes. In a study of 500 adults presenting to a primary care walk-in clinic with a physical symptom, researchers used scoring of 38 physicians on the Physician's Belief Scale and their perception of encounter difficulty using the Difficult Doctor-Patient Relationship Questionnaire. They found that patients presenting with physical symptoms who are perceived as difficult are more likely to have a depressive or anxiety disorder, poorer functional status, unmet expectations, reduced satisfaction, and greater use of health care services. Although not definitively studied, physician characteristics associated with difficult encounters appear to be the psychosocial factors the physician is experiencing, either job related (burnout, job dissatisfaction, or stress) or personal (depression or anxiety).[3] It appears that when designing safe systems, staff self-awareness should be considered as part of the human factors that can affect perceptions and consequent communication. Communication skills, including self-assessment, should be included in patient safety training.

There are a number of ways to improve communication in the ambulatory health care setting. These involve improving systemic policies, including training staff in understanding and monitoring the workplace and staff behaviors where human factors may be affecting those systems, and assessing for workarounds and risk points for communication breakdowns.

Human Factors Affect Good Communication

An initial step is to learn how human factors affect an organization's established systems and processes and can contribute to health care delivery complexity. Impairment of short-term memory, negative effects of stress, fatigue, multitasking, interruptions, and distractions are a few of these human factors—all of which influence communication. Improving the policies and processes regarding communication in vital areas for maintaining quality and safety requires a collaborative effort between all disciplines of the health care team.

People Communicate Differently

One important finding over the past several years has been the appreciation of the vast difference in communication styles between clinic staff and physicians. Patients and providers communicate differently as well. A culture of safety bridges the gaps of communication between groups and individuals to prevent communication-related errors and barriers to quality care. As James Reason, safety guru, has said, a culture of safety creates a safe experience of shared values and beliefs.[4] The SBAR technique featured in Chapter 7, "Staff Education and Training," is an example of a tool that has been adopted widely to bridge this gap in communication styles.

Tools for Improving Communication

Exemplary tools for understanding and improving communication and collaboration include the Safety Attitudes Questionnaires and Human Factors Training Modules. These tools focus on briefings, assertiveness, situational awareness, and debriefings. Other models will be mentioned in this chapter and throughout the book.

Organization and Communication

Adverse events and potential adverse events occur when systems break down. Three areas that have been shown to represent an inordinate number of errors are those related to filing, transitions of care, and telephone and other verbal orders.

Filing System Errors

In one series of studies of the data analyzed by staff of family medicine practices in the United States and other countries, filing system error in the United States was the third highest type of error cited. Errors in filing that can contribute to patient safety risks include lost or

misplaced files or test results, filing reports in the wrong chart, and using the wrong patient chart in the office.[5]

As Dovey et al. state in their 2003 article in *American Family Physician*, of 416 error reports filed by U.S. family physicians in two medical error studies in 2000 and 2001, 30% of the proposed solutions related to improving mechanisms of communication.[5] Specific, practical suggestions to change habits included stopping the use of carbon copy prescription forms, doing urgent lab tests in the office, and using flagging systems to draw attention to information needing action. Various double-checking systems were also favored.

When searching for solutions to medical errors, asking those involved in providing care for their ideas may be a rewarding strategy. Best practices for proper filing involve standardization of the following:

- Types of files, shapes, colors, labels
- Formatting of files
- Process used for filing such that it becomes habitual
- Method of sign-offs
- Methodology of nonsoftware filing systems on every person's computer
- Forced functions built into software systems such that filing something incorrectly will be immediately noticed and intercepted.

Coordination of Care in Transition Points/ Handoff Communications

Coordinating care at transition points, sometimes referred to as "handoffs," is integral to continuity of care.[6] This continuity includes communicating medications that the patient is taking, prescribed or recommended follow-up care, and referral process and information sharing with other providers. Joint Commission requirements call for implementing a standardized approach to handoff communications, including providing to the patient an opportunity to ask and respond to questions.

In a study of five primary care practices, transition of care was named as one factor responsible for adverse events. These events were classified as to actual or potential harm to patients using a multilevel taxonomy of cognitive and system factors.[7] A total of 78 reports were relevant to patient safety and analyzable, including 21 adverse events (27%) and 50 near misses (64%). Most reports referenced administrative errors; the most frequent contributing factor was faulty work organization, identified in 71 events. These included excessive task demands and fragmentation of care; in other words, unclear policies covered situations of transition of care.

In another example, a study of primary care in the Netherlands found that a mix of methods is needed to identify adverse events.[8] General practitioners used a variety of types of reports, including physician-reported adverse events, pharmacist-reported adverse events, patients' experiences of adverse events, assessment of a random sample of medical records, and assessment of all deceased patients. A total of 68 events were identified using these methods. The patient survey accounted for the highest number of events, the pharmacist reports for the lowest number, and, interestingly, there were no individual events reported by more than one method.

In ambulatory settings, patients may receive care from a number of different clinicians and facilities; however, one physician practice will hold the principal responsibility for coordinating the patient's care across time and space. That practice often uses a combination of paper-based, verbal, and electronic communication methods during the course of care. It takes planning to coordinate and track a patient's clinical care. It is important to standardize a process for handing off patients to other caregivers.

A list of items that should be considered when maintaining good handoff techniques is presented as a self-assessment tool in Table 2-1, page 16.

Telephone and Verbal Orders

The Institute for Safe Medical Practices reports a case of a patient with a bladder infection. His physician called in a prescription for the antibiotic Noroxin (norfloxacin). But the pharmacist thought the order was for Neurontin (gabapentin), a medication used to treat seizures. Fortunately, the patient read the medication leaflet stapled to his medication bag, noticed the drug he received is used to treat seizures, and asked the pharmacist about it.

Verbal orders have great potential for error, particularly with medications. Although use of fax, e-mail, and point-of-care computer programs may reduce the need to communicate orders by voice, the need for verbal orders will never be entirely eliminated.

✓ **Joint Commission requirements call for establishing a plan for the use of verbal or telephone orders or for telephone reporting of critical test results. The individual giving the order should verify the complete order or test result by having the receiving person record and "read back" the complete information.**

Whenever possible, medical orders (particularly medication orders) and reports of critical test results should be in writing. Problems in verbal orders that could increase the risk to patient safety include the following[9]:

■ Mentioning multiple medications at once
■ Differences of dialect, accents, pronunciation
■ Distractions and sound muffling such as background noise
■ Unfamiliar terms. Drug names may be particularly difficult to understand and repeat.
■ Drug names can sound alike (*see* "Look-Alike/Sound-Alike Medications," pages 43–44 in Chapter 3)
■ Communicating lab values. Many of these types of errors involve misinterpretation of blood sugar levels.
■ Miscommunication of information regarding patient diagnoses, comorbid conditions, and current medication list (medication reconciliation).
■ Staff members who do not write down the order first, or perform safety checks such as read-backs and two checks (*see* "Tool: Two Checks," below, and "Tool: Read-Backs," on page 19) before relaying that information to another person or using that information directly in patient care.

- -

TOOL: Two Checks

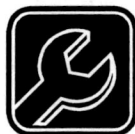

Performing two checks helps to verify and provide clear and accurate information. This is particularly imperative when identifying patients and preparing medications (*see* Chapter 1, "Patient-Centered Care"). Make sure the clinical staff or physician confirms the patient's identity before he or she administers any medication or treatment. Common identifiers include the patient's name, birth date, and social security or other identification number.

- -

Table 2-1. Assessment of Hand-off (Transition) Practices

Ask the following questions when your practice transfers responsibility for the care of a patient to another physician, practice, or institution:

- Does the practice identify the clinician responsible for accepting the patient?
- Does the practice confirm that the clinician receives and accepts responsibility for the patient?
- Do you have a method to confirm that necessary clinical information about the patient is transmitted to the accepting clinician?
- Does the practice have a way to determine that the information was received?
- Do you document in the patient's medical record that the patient has been transferred and that responsibility has been accepted by the receiving clinician, practice, or other institution?

When a patient is referred to an outside pathology laboratory, or a patient's specimen is sent to an outside pathology laboratory, does the practice do the following:

- Track the testing process, including the following:
  —When the patient is referred?
  —When the specimen is sent?
  —To what laboratory the patient or specimen is sent?
  —The test(s) to be performed?
  —When a report is expected?
  —Which clinicians in the practice and outside the practice are to receive the report?
- Ensure and document in the patient's medical record that the report has been received by the practice?
- Document that the report has been delivered to the designated clinician(s)?
- Document that the clinician(s) is informed if a report has *not* been received by the expected date?
- Have a standardized mechanism to contact the pathology laboratory when reports are not received by the expected date?

When a patient is admitted to a hospital, nursing home, home care agency, rehabilitation center, and so on, does the practice do the following:

- Maintain a process to communicate all medications (name, dose, frequency, route, and purpose) that a patient is receiving?
- Have a process to communicate other important patient information, including relevant history, preferences, family/living situation, and so forth?

When a patient is sent to another physician or practice for consultation, does the practice do the following:

- Track the consultation, including the following:
  —When the referral for consultation is made?
  —To which consulting physician/practice?
  —The purpose of the consultation?
  —When a report is expected?
  —Which clinicians in the practice and outside the

practice are to receive the report?

- Ensure and document in the patient's medical record that the following is done:
  —The consultation report is received by the practice?
  —The consultation is delivered to the specified clinician(s)?
  —The practice informs the specified clinician(s) if a report has not been received by the expected time?
- Have a mechanism to contact the consulting physician/practice when reports are not received by the expected date?

- Does the practice have a standardized way to determine which laboratory, pathology, and imaging test results are to be considered "critical"?
- Does the practice have a mechanism that is distinct from the routine process for the following:
  —Handling test results?
  —Determining when a critical test result is received?
  —Immediately delivering that result to an appropriate clinician(s)?
  —Delivering, when appropriate, to the patient?
- Does the mechanism for disseminating critical or emergent test results to clinicians and patients also function outside normal business hours?
- Does the practice track the following:
  —When and to what imaging facility each patient is sent?
  —The test(s) to be performed?
  —When a report is expected?
  —Whether that report is received as expected?
  —Which clinician(s) in the practice will receive the report?
- Does the practice ensure that the imaging test report:
  —Is received by the practice?
  —Is delivered to the specified clinician(s)?
  —Informs the specified clinician(s) if a report has not been received by the expected time?
- Does the practice document the results and their receipt in the patient's medical record?
- Does the practice have a mechanism to contact the imaging facility when reports are not received by the expected date?
- Are the results of laboratory, pathology, and imaging tests communicated to the patient in a timely manner (24 to 48 hours)?
- Does the practice confirm and document that the patient received the results?
- Are patients notified of all laboratory, pathology, and imaging test results, including those that are "negative," whether or not they require further clinical action?
- Does the practice provide all patients with easy access to their consultative, laboratory, imaging, and other results?
- Are all patients educated on how to obtain this information?

Source: Modified from *The Physician Practice Patient Safety Assessment*. Institute for Safe Medication Practices, Health Research and Educational Trust, and Medical Group Management Association, 2005.

**Table 2-2. NCC MERP Recommendations to Reduce Medication Errors
Associated with Verbal Medication Orders and Prescriptions**

1. Verbal communication of prescription or medication orders should be limited to urgent situations where immediate written or electronic communication is not feasible.
2. Health care organizations should establish policies and procedures that do the following:
   - Describe limitations or prohibitions on use of verbal orders
   - Provide a mechanism to ensure validity/authenticity of the prescriber
   - List the elements required for inclusion in a complete verbal order
   - Describe situations in which verbal orders may be used
   - List and define the individuals who may send and receive verbal orders
   - Provide guidelines for clear and effective communication of verbal orders
3. Leaders of health care organizations should promote a culture in which it is acceptable, and strongly encouraged, for staff to question prescribers when any questions or disagreements about verbal orders arise. Questions about verbal orders should be resolved prior to preparing, or dispensing, or administering the medication.
4. Verbal orders for antineoplastic agents should NOT be permitted under any circumstances. These medications are not administered in emergency or urgent situations, and they have a narrow margin of safety.
5. Elements that should be included in a verbal order include the following:
   - Name of patient
   - Age and weight of patient, when appropriate
   - Drug name
   - Dosage form (for example, tablets, capsules, inhalants)
   - Exact strength or concentration
   - Dose, frequency, and route
   - Quantity and/or duration
   - Purpose or indication (unless disclosure is considered inappropriate by the prescriber)
   - Specific instructions for use
   - Name of prescriber, and telephone number when appropriate
   - Name of individual transmitting the order, if different from the prescriber
6. The content of verbal orders should be clearly communicated:
   - The name of the drug should be confirmed by any of the following:
     —Spelling
     —Providing both the brand and generic names of the medication
     —Providing the indication for use
   - To avoid confusion with spoken numbers, a dose such as 50 mg should be dictated as "fifty milligrams . . . five zero milligrams" to distinguish from "fifteen milligrams . . . one five milligrams."
   - To avoid confusion with drug name modifiers, such as prefixes and suffixes, additional spelling-assistance methods should be used (that is, "S as in Sam," "X as in x-ray").
   - Instructions for use should be provided without abbreviations. For example, "1 tab TID" should be communicated as "Take/give one tablet three times daily."
   - Whenever possible, the receiver of the order should write down the complete order to enter it into a computer, then read it back, and receive confirmation from the individual who gave the order or test result.
7. All verbal orders should be reduced immediately to writing and signed by the individual receiving the order.
8. Verbal orders should be documented in the patient's medical record, reviewed, and countersigned by the prescriber as soon as possible.

Source: National Coordinating Council for Medication Error Reporting and Prevention: *Recommendations to Reduce Medication Errors Associated with Verbal Medication Orders and Prescriptions*, Feb. 24, 2006. http://www.nccmerp.org/council/council2001-02-20.html (accessed Mar. 8, 2009).

Effective policies and procedures for the use of verbal orders include the following[10]:

- Describe limitations or prohibitions on the use of verbal orders.
- Provide a mechanism for the recipient to ensure validity/authenticity of the prescriber.
- List the required elements of a complete verbal order.
- Describe situations in which verbal orders may or may not be used.
- List and define the individuals who may send and receive verbal orders.
- Provide guidelines for clear and effective communication of verbal orders.

Table 2-2, above, includes recommendations from the National Coordinating Council for Medication Error Reporting and Prevention to reduce medication errors associated with verbal medication orders and pre-

Sidebar 2-1. Sample Policy Related to Verbal Telephone Orders

This document is not meant to be used "as is" and is only shared as an example of the kind of policy you might want to implement in your facility. Because different types of facilities have different requirements and staffing, there is no "one size fits all" policy statement related to verbal orders. We suggest that you consult with your legal counsel and clinical managers in developing this or any policy or procedure.

Purpose

To reduce errors associated with misinterpreted verbal or telephone communications of medication orders or test results.

Policy

1. Verbal communication of prescription or medication orders and test results is limited to urgent situations in which immediate written or electronic communication is not feasible.
2. Verbal orders and test results are not allowed when the prescriber is present and the patient's medical record is available, except during a sterile procedure or in an emergency situation, in which case a repeat-back is acceptable.
3. Verbal orders are not permitted for nonformulary drugs, except during a sterile procedure or in an emergency situation, in which case a repeat-back is acceptable.
4. Verbal orders are not permitted for chemotherapy.
5. Verbal orders and test results are not permitted via voice mail.
6. The following job categories are authorized to give verbal orders: [include list]
7. The following job categories are authorized to accept verbal orders: [include list]

Procedures

1. Verbal orders and test results, when allowed, will be immediately written down by the recipient, read back by the recipient, and confirmed or corrected by the prescriber. The order must be written before it is read back.
2. Both parties will pronounce numerical digits separately—saying, for example, "one six" instead of "sixteen."
3. For medication orders, the prescriber will spell the name of any unfamiliar medication, if either party feels this is necessary.
4. For medication orders, prescribers will include the purpose of the drug to ensure that the order makes sense in the context of the patient's condition.
5. For medication orders, both parties will include the mg/kg dose along with the patient's specific dose for all verbal neonatal/pediatric medication orders.
6. For medication orders, both parties will express doses of medications by unit of weight (for example, mg, g, mEq, mMol).
7. The recipient will record each verbal order directly onto an order sheet in the patient's medical record and will include phone or pager numbers in case it is necessary for follow-up questions.
8. Recipients of verbal orders will sign, date, time, and note the order at the time it is written on the order sheet or entered into the computer system.
9. Prescribers will verify, sign, and date orders within ___ hours.
10. Pharmacy will disallow medication requests from nursing units to the pharmacy unless the verbal order has been transcribed onto an order form and simultaneously faxed or otherwise seen by a pharmacist before the medication is dispensed.
11. Verbal orders, when spoken and when transcribed, will use only approved abbreviations.
12. Verbal medication orders will include the following information:
    12.1. Date and time order is received
    12.2. Patient name
    12.3. Drug name (brand or generic)
    12.4. Dosage form (for example, tablets, capsules, inhalants, and so on)
    12.5. Strength or concentration
    12.6. Dose
    12.7. Frequency
    12.8. Route
    12.9. Quantity and/or duration
    12.10. Name of prescriber
    12.11. Signature of order recipient

Source: ECRI Institute and Institute for Safe Medication Practices: Improving the safety of telephone or verbal orders. *PA-PSRS Patient Safety Advisory* 3:1–6, Jun. 2006. http://www.psa.state.pa.us/ADVISORIES/AdvisoryLibrary/2006/June3(2)/Pages/01b.aspx (last accessed Sep. 22, 2009.)

Table 2-3. Key Words to Improve Communication		
Discontinuation	**Causes**	**Unique phrases**
D/C	Because [b/c]	Stopped taking
Not [been] tak[ing]	Due	Not [n't] tolerable
Stopped	Secon[dary] [to]	Unable to tolerate
Switched		

Source: Cantor M.N., Feldman H.J., Triola M.M.: Using trigger phrases to detect adverse drug reactions in ambulatory care notes. *Qual Saf Health Care* 16:132–134, Apr. 2007.

scriptions. Use the list as a self-assessment for verbal orders in your organization. The Pennsylvania Patient Safety Authority designed a sample policy for reciting verbal orders presented in Sidebar 2-1, page 18.

TOOL: Read-Backs

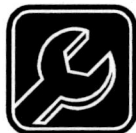

Read-backs and repeat-backs for verbal orders have proven to help protect safety regarding communicating medications or instructions, particularly those instructions that involve drug names or numbers.[6] Take the following steps to improve clarity in handoff messages[6]:

1. Hear the message. Keep the patient's safety in mind as you listen.
2. Write down the message.
3. Read back the message. Spell out troublesome words.
4. Ask for confirmation that the message was received correctly.

TIPS

- Medication order recipients should repeat the name of the drug and dosage order to the prescriber and request or provide correct spelling, using aids such as "B as in ball," "M as in Mary." All numbers should be spelled out; for example, 16 should be stated as "one six" to avoid confusion with the number 60.

- Avoid using abbreviations. For example, "1 tab TID" should be stated as "Take/give one tablet three times daily." (For more information, including the list of do-not-use abbreviations, *see* Chapter 3, "Medication Use.")

- Be specific when talking about look-alike/sound-alike drugs.

Standardized terminology, that is, key words, used in medical records and notes has been shown to be effective in identifying breakdowns in communication. In the medicine clinic at Bellevue Hospital in 2003–2004, researchers devised a lexicon of trigger phrases to detect adverse drug reactions (ADRs) in ambulatory care notes, a vital component of care transitions.[11] Outpatient ADRs have been estimated to contribute to between 3.2% and 6.5% of hospital admissions, and in one study, to 4% of hospital readmissions. The researchers devised an automated system for detecting ADRs, which was successful at detecting medication discontinuation and other changes to medication regimens. Study results show that an automated system can detect potential ADRs with moderate sensitivity and high specificity and has the potential to serve as the basis for a larger-scale reporting system. The lexicon used in this study is shown in Table 2-3, above. These "trigger phrases" relate to the discontinuation of or noncompliance with prescription medications, and could be used by an AHC organization in its own assessment of care notes to identify and address potential ADRs.

Laboratory and Test Results

Joint Commission requirements call for measuring, assessing, and, if needed, taking action to improve the timeliness of reporting and the timeliness of receipt of critical tests. Requirements also include the review of critical results and values by the responsible licensed caregiver.

A key area for improving patient safety is the laboratory, whether that laboratory is external to the ambulatory setting or a part of it. According to the 2002 National Ambulatory Medical Care Survey, the average family physician orders laboratory testing in 29% of the patients he or she sees, and internists order tests after 38% of patient encounters.[12] Imaging studies are ordered in 10% and 12% of encounters, respectively.[13]

The processes of laboratory testing and lab results involve complex systems in which risks exist and errors can occur. Even when tests are ordered, processed, and returned to the practice correctly, the decision-making process prompted by these test results can be complex. An estimated 15% to 54% of errors in primary care reported by primary care practices are related to the testing process.[13]

Despite the importance of these decisions, physicians often manage these results in the midst of a busy practice day, between patient visits. The adverse consequences of administrative errors in testing processes include missed or delayed diagnoses, duplication of services, unnecessary or delayed interventions, patient dissatisfaction, and litigation.[13]

The Testing Process

Everyone involved in any of the processes, including ordering tests, collecting and transporting specimens, testing specimens, reporting results, and reacting to results, can affect patient outcomes and patient safety. For ambulatory care, organizations should assess contract reference laboratories using the timeliness expectation criteria outlined in the written contract. They should also assess internal reporting against organization policies relating to timely reporting of critical values for those tests being performed in-house.

The various stages of laboratory testing are classified as preanalytic, analytic, and postanalytic, which helps determine where errors are most likely to occur in the testing process. Most laboratory errors originate in the pre- and postanalytic phases. Potential problems that could impact communication and patient safety include the following.[1,13]

Preanalytic Processes: These processes are structured around ordering and implementing the test. Problems might include a test requisition system that is not user friendly or test names and abbreviations that might be confusing.
- Inadequate patient preparation could provide questionable results if the test is performed or could require delay in patient testing until the preparation is appropriate.
- Specimen collection and processing might include errors such as improper patient identification and

labeling, improper use of appropriate blood containers for requested tests, and mixing specimens that are anticoagulated.

Analytic Processes: These processes involve conducting the test. Of the three phases, this is the least problematic, due to the implementation of regulatory requirements in the past several years. However, error frequency still ranges between 4% and 32%, and point-of-care testing has a higher frequency than in traditional laboratory settings[14] (*see* Chapter 7, "Staff Education and Training").

Although the term *bedside testing* has traditionally been associated with inpatient care, this term actually involves care given anywhere in any health care organization, including the ambulatory setting, that is not under direct control of laboratory management. For this reason, organizations are still responsible for ensuring that those performing point-of-care testing are properly trained and supervised and that policies and procedures covering all units and areas of a clinic are consistent with each other and with good professional practice.[15]

Postanalytic Processes: These processes are structured around tracking and returning the test, responding to and documenting results, notifying a patient of results, and following up with needed action.[1,13] At this stage, results are reported and interpreted. Error frequency estimates range from 9% to 55%. Issues that need to be addressed in reporting critical values include the following:
- Calling the result to someone who can take action
- Linking the patient at all times to a responsible physician
- Documenting full information: patient name, test, value, date, time, reporter, and receiver
- Requiring acknowledgment of receipt of the report
- Having a clearly understood backup system and avoiding a chain of reporting using a central call system
- Agreeing on which test results require communication
- Using the same policy across all settings and domains

Clearly planned and well-thought-out systems of communication are the most effective way of ensuring patient safety regarding testing, as shown in Figure 2-1, page 21. The patient must be notified of testing results, whether good or bad. Access Community Health Care in Chicago tackled these issies in a project described in

Figure 2-1. Error-Free Testing Process

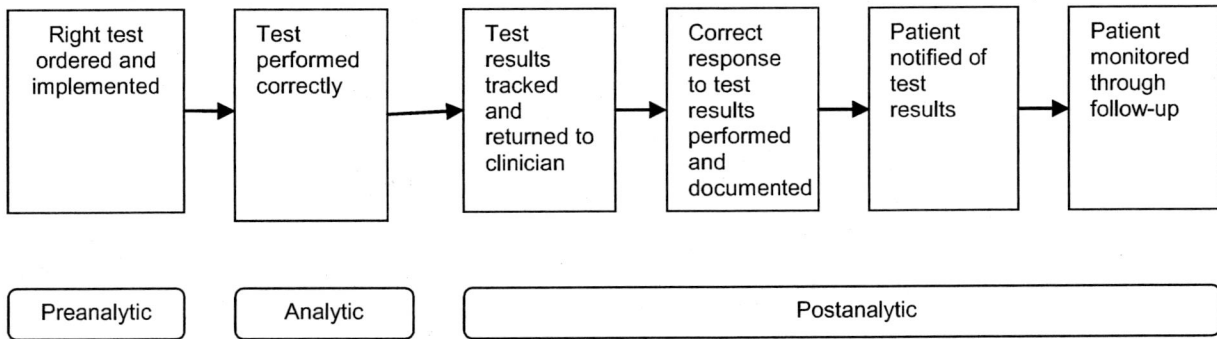

| Right test ordered and implemented | → | Test performed correctly | → | Test results tracked and returned to clinician | → | Correct response to test results performed and documented | → | Patient notified of test results | → | Patient monitored through follow-up |

| Preanalytic | Analytic | Postanalytic |

In an effective, practical system, the testing process occurs in an orderly, error-free manner, as shown.

Source: Hickner J.M., et al.: Issues and initiatives in the testing process in primary care physician offices. In Schiff G.D. (ed.): *Getting Results: Reliably Communicating and Acting on Critical Test Results.* Oakbrook Terrace, IL: Joint Commission Resources, 2006, pp. 31–41.

Figure 2-2. Sample of a Simple Process Map

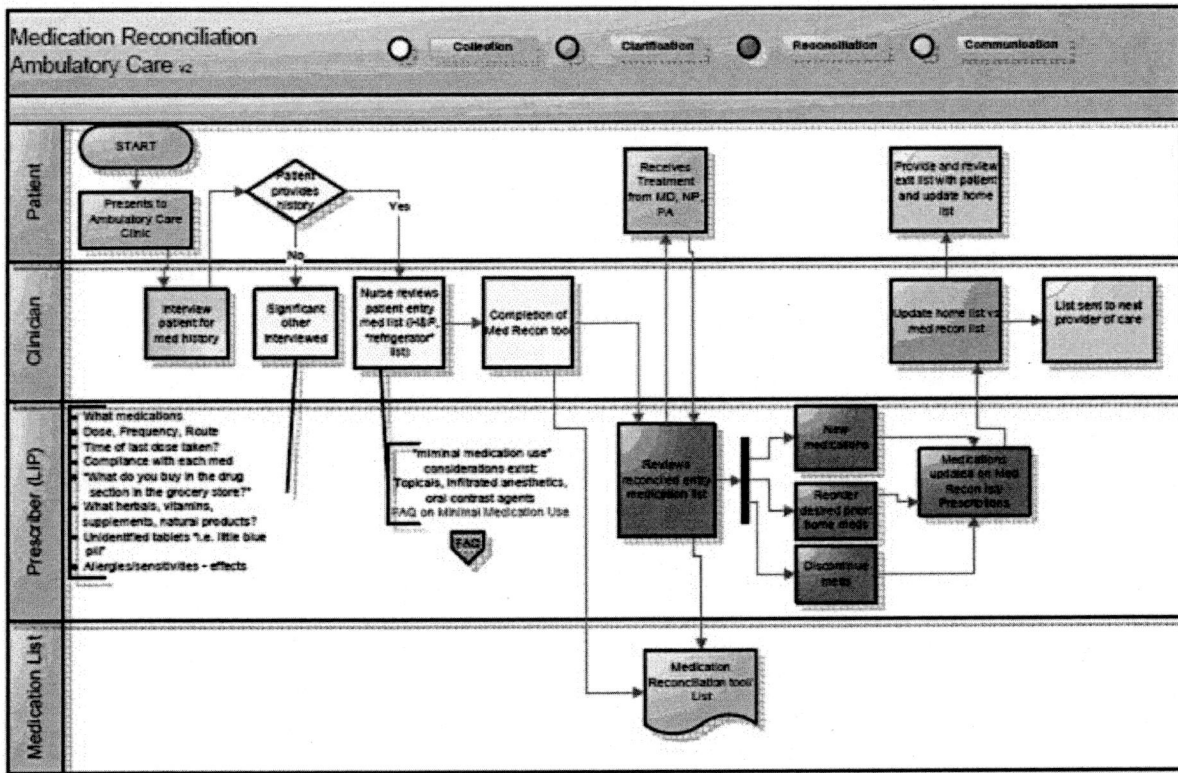

Simple mapping of a process can help staff determine safety risks.

Source: Gary J. Robb, R.Ph., M.B.A., C.B.B., Consultant, Joint Commission Resources, Oak Brook, IL.

Table 2-4. Suggested Interventions to Improve Test-Process Management

Ordering and Implementing Tests
- Standardize one method for collecting, preparing, and delivering specimens to outside facilities.
- Standardize how patients, billing providers, and ordering providers are identified on laboratory requisition forms. Work with suppliers to create forms and protocols that fit a particular practice's needs.
- Confirm that correct procedure was followed before the patient leaves the office.
- Design a system to double-check patient identification, tube labeling, and correct order form.
- Use a checklist for clinician sign-off on tests ordered, specimens drawn, reagent tube used, and so on.

Tracking and Returning Tests
- Standardize how test results will be communicated from the laboratory to the practice. Variation in how laboratories report results increases potential for error. Use compulsively one method to record when tests are requested, completed, sent, and received.
- Create a backup, fail-safe system to doubly reinforce error prevention. Some practices use a dual tracking system, perhaps using a technician, or paper based and electronic.

Response and Documentation of Information
- Primary care physicians and staff report that 7% of all testing process errors are related to incorrect, delayed, or inappropriate clinician responses to test results.
- Clinicians should create a system for receiving test results, deciding on the appropriate action, and documenting the plan of action in the medical record.
- An electronic test tracking system integrated into an electronic medical record is best but not accessible to all practices. Other methods might include date stamping physician's notes onto the test results form and inserting the notes into the patient record after a copy is mailed to the patient. Staff can brainstorm systems that work in an individual practice.

Patient Notification
- Instruct patients to expect to be contacted regarding their test results within a certain range of time. Patients can be encouraged to serve as their own safeguard for their care; if they do not hear within a certain amount of time, they should call the office. Patients may believe that "no news is good news"; however, *this method is not reliable as a backup.*
- Design a method to confirm that patients have been notified, such as an auto-generated letter and telephone system.
- The overall process of logging test results can also keep track of when a copy of the tests results, a brief explanation of the test's purpose, and a written note from the physician are sent to the patient. Handwriting must be clear; a patient receiving an illegible note can find no information or comfort.

Source: Modified from Hickner J.M., et al.: Issues and initiatives in the testing process in primary care physician offices. In Schiff G.D. (ed.): *Getting Results: Reliably Communicating and Acting on Critical Test Results.* Oakbrook Terrace, IL: Joint Commission Resources, 2006, pp. 31–41.

---

the case study beginning on page 26.

Causes of Errors in the Testing Process

Laboratory and clinical staff should work together to establish and practice communication systems in which no bit of data or information can fall through the cracks. Backup systems and delta checks (when test results vary from what the patient has tested historically) are imperative.

Causes of errors can include difficulty contacting patients, time constraints, and physician forgetfulness. Hickner et al. identified the following four factors as

contributing to errors[13]:
1. Inadequate office systems
2. Inadequate oversight of those systems
3. Inadequate training of staff in the policies
4. Procedures associated with laboratory test management, and lack of physician awareness of the frequency of errors

Barriers and Factors That Contribute to Laboratory Test Errors

Physicians and staff in a family practice conducted 18 focus groups with 139 participants to identify errors and their contributing factors. The most commonly reported contributing factors included not following procedures, lack of standardization, and inadequate systems and communication. Cultural barriers included personal resistance to change, lack of buy-in from staff or providers, and no perceived consequences. Cultural barriers were seen as much harder to overcome than process-related barriers. The most frequently mentioned desired improvements were technology and additional staff; interestingly, the study authors noted, these were *not* related to the most commonly named contributing factors.

Improving test management involves excellent communication and organization. Fewer than one fifth of internists and family physicians have instituted adequate systems to monitor the flow of laboratory tests they order.[16] Unfortunately, specific interventions to improve test-process management have not been fully studied or designed, but some suggestions are presented in Table 2-4, page 22.

Follow-Up

A medical practice cannot track adherence to all medical recommendations, but abnormal test results must have a system for tracking. These results must be communicated in a timely manner, clearly and succinctly, and must employ means for ensuring that the communication is complete and accurate.

Automated alert systems and computerized results managers linked to integrated electronic medical records may be a promising system to decrease the number of delays, but in practices without this resource, other simpler but just as clear mechanisms must be devised.

Tracking critical test results is an important contributor to diagnostic delays. Delayed diagnoses can lead to improper treatment and are therefore risks for patient safety. Diagnostic errors are rarely on the radar screen even in the patient safety community.[17] Examples of successful interventions for tracking lab test results are presented in Sidebar 2-2, page 24.

Challenges for Imaging

The field of advanced imaging technology has made impressive strides, leading to major enhancements in a physician's ability to diagnose a variety of diseases. As the capacity for imaging tests has increased, so have the challenges for patient safety. These challenges are discussed in Chapter 6, "Environment and Equipment," and a related case study is presented in Chapter 7, "Staff Education and Training," beginning on page 122.

TOOL: Simple Process Mapping

The processes, or steps, that yield successful imaging and results are numerous and require close review to identify risk point and inefficiencies. One tool to help with that is process mapping. Process mapping is a way to determine where bottlenecks, delays, and wasted space and time reside in any health care process. A process map, this one for medication reconciliation, is shown in Figure 2-2, page 21. (Medication reconciliation is discussed in detail in Chapter 3 beginning on page 44.)

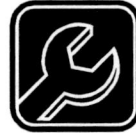

Steps in process mapping are as follows:
- Define the objectives, scope (start and end points for the process you are studying), and focus for the process mapping workshop.
- Meet with managerial, clinical, and service leaders beforehand so that they feel involved in the process. Use these meetings to agree to the scope that you will work on and the three or four basic steps that you will explore in detail at the workshop.
- Identify the staff groups that are involved at each step in the journey. Include clinical, managerial, administrative, and support staff—the people who actually deliver the process.
- Organize about a half-day event to draw the map and a half day to analyze and look for improvement opportunities. You can run these together as a full-day event or as two half days but not more than two weeks apart.
- Arrange a suitable venue, preferably off site because this provides a neutral setting and people are less likely to be interrupted.

Allow plenty of time for setting up the workshop, at least an hour before the planned start time of the event. Ask one of the lead clinicians to open the event, and use an independent facilitator not connected with the pathway. A roll of brown paper or wallpaper can be fixed firmly to the wall. Use sticky notes to write in the steps in the process so you can stick them to the background, but move them around if you need to squeeze in extra steps. You will also

---

Sidebar 2-2. Examples of Successful Testing Follow-Up Interventions

Methods that have been used to track critical and abnormal test results include the following:

1. To track notifications and follow-up regarding abnormal Papinicolou (Pap) smears, one Australian primary care practice attached a patient education tear-off sheet to the test results.[1]

2. One organization implemented a number of changes to its laboratory test process. Tips from its findings include the following[2]:

   - Prelabel requisition forms with the agency's logo and telephone number.
   - Install a clipboard at the test requisition drop box where drop-off and pick-up times are recorded. Clinical staff sign the board when they leave a specimen, also noting the patient identifier. The courier signs the board at every interaction.
   - Instruct the receptionist to no longer take the laboratory value(s) by phone but instead have the lab fax the results to the home care department and call a few minutes beforehand to alert that department to look out for the results.
   - Select a few clinical staff within the organization to handle those calls, faxes, and reports.
   - Ensure that all laboratory results are deposited into a designated LAB mailbox located near the fax machine.
   - Institute a schedule to replace fax paper three times each day.
   - Synchronize all clinical staff's voice mails to a scripted message such as, "Hello, this is Jane Smith, L.P.N. If you are calling with a critical laboratory value, please press zero for immediate help."

3. Communication was seen to be at the root of an investigation of timeliness or reporting laboratory values. Moore et al., with the Division of General Internal Medicine at Mount Sinai School of Medicine in New York, studied the timeliness of follow-up with outpatient test results.[3] They examined the management of markedly elevated serum potassium test results, a process which has been shown to be associated with 22% of reported medical errors in the ambulatory setting. For one year (2003–2004), the researchers reviewed the medical records of all patients seen in a large primary care practice, with serum potassium levels greater than or equal to 5.8 mEq/L.

   In almost 13,000 serum potassium tests performed, there were 109 cases of the criterion level in 86 patients. Although more than half of patients had been recalled to the clinic for repeat testing, one quarter of patients had no repeat tests until they were seen at routine follow-up visits. Those patients over age 65 had a lower likelihood of having repeat testing within one week. Variability was seen at two critical points in the transmission of information:

   1. First, from the laboratory to an attending physician
   2. Second, the time it takes for the patient to be contacted after the physician is notified about the critical laboratory result

   The process was evaluated as lacking standardization. After receiving the results, the physician had four options for follow-up:

   1. Contact the patient directly to arrange the recommended follow-up.
   2. Request that the clinical staff make the arrangements.
   3. Hand off the responsibility for making arrangements to another physician.
   4. Take no action.

References

1. Mitchell H., Medley G.: Notification of Pap smear results. A Victorian survey. *Aust Fam Physician* 27 (Suppl. 1):S7–S10, Jan. 1998.
2. Lochridge K.: Do you know where your critical lab values are? Communication of critical lab results. *Home Healthc Nurse* 24:121–125, Feb. 2006.
3. Moore C.R., et al.: Follow-up of markedly elevated serum potassium results in the ambulatory setting: Implications for patient safety. *Am J Med Qual* 21:115–124, Mar.–Apr. 2006.

---

need at least one flipchart and several markers.

Start by mapping some main headings on the wallpaper, such as the "high level" steps in the process: that is, "presenting symptoms," "referral," "diagnosis," "patient," and so forth. This will remind people that the purpose of the event is to map the whole of the journey, not just the elements with which they are familiar. Focus the discussion on identifying the steps in the process. If other problems or issues arise, or there are problems that cannot be resolved in the moment, keep a flipchart ready to "park" these, to be addressed later. Agree on the next steps before closing the workshop.

References

1. The Joint Commission: *Engaging Physicians in Patient Safety: A Handbook for Leaders.* Oakbrook Terrace, IL: Joint Commission Resources, 2006.

2. Jackson J.L., Kroenke K.: Difficult patient encounters in the ambulatory clinic: Clinical predictors and outcomes. *Arch Intern Med* 159:1069–1075, May 24, 1999.

3. Kroenke K.: Unburdening the difficult clinical encounter. *Arch Intern Med* 169:333–334, Feb. 23, 2009.

4. Chenot T.M.: Patient safety and the ambulatory care setting. *Northeast FL Med* 58:23–26, Fall 2007.

5. Dovey S.M., et al.: Family physicians' solutions to common medical errors. *Am Fam Physician* 67:1168, Mar. 15, 2003.

6. The Joint Commission: *Improving Hand-Off Communication.* Oakbrook Terrace, IL: Joint Commission Resources, 2007.

7. Kostopoulou O., Delaney B.: Confidential reporting of patient safety events in primary care: Results from a multilevel classification of cognitive and system factors. *Qual Saf Health Care* 16:95–100, Apr. 2007.

8. Wetzels R., et al.: Mix of methods is needed to identify adverse events in general practice: A prospective observational study. *BMC Fam Pract* 9:35–39, Jun. 15, 2008.

9. ECRI Institute & Institute for Safe Medication Practices: Improving the safety of telephone or verbal orders. *PA-PSRS Patient Safety Advisory* 3:1–6, Jun. 2006. http://www.psa.state.pa.us/ADVISORIES/AdvisoryLibrary/2006/Jun3(2)/Pages/01.aspx (accessed Feb. 20, 2009).

10. National Coordinating Council for Medication Error Reporting and Prevention: *Recommendations to Reduce Medication Errors Associated with Verbal Medication Orders and Prescriptions.* Feb. 24, 2006. http://www.nccmerp.org/ council/council2001-02-20.html (accessed Mar. 8, 2009).

11. Cantor M.N., Feldman H.J., Triola M.M.: Using trigger phrases to detect adverse drug reactions in ambulatory care notes. *Qual Saf Health Care* 16:132–134, Apr. 2007.

12. Woodwell D.A., Cherry D.K.: National Ambulatory Medical Care Survey: 2002 summary. *Adv Data* 346:1–44, Aug. 26, 2004.

13. Hickner J.M., et al.: Issues and initiatives in the testing process in primary care physician offices. In Schiff G.D. (ed.): *Getting Results: Reliably Communicating and Acting on Critical Test Results.* Oakbrook Terrace, IL: Joint Commission Resources, 2006.

14. Bonini P., et al.: Errors in laboratory medicine. *Clin Chem* 48:691–698, May 1, 2002.

15. Pasternak D.P.: Bedside (Point-of-Care) testing in hospitals: The Joint Commission international perspective. *Point of Care: The Journal of Near-Patient Testing & Technology* 7:233–238, Dec. 2008.

16. Boohaker E.A., et al.: Patient notification and follow-up of abnormal test results: A physician survey. *Arch Intern Med* 156:327–331, Feb. 12, 1996.

17. Graber M.: Diagnostic errors in medicine: A case of neglect. In Schiff G.D. (ed.): *Getting Results: Reliably Communicating and Acting on Critical Test Results.* Oakbrook Terrace, IL: Joint Commission Resources, 2006.

Case Study: The Testing Process

CASE STUDY AT A GLANCE

Organization: Access Community Health Network

Setting: Network of 50 sites in the Chicago metropolitan area, each site a recognized Federally Qualified Health Center

Patient Safety Topic: Safety and quality of the testing process

Accomplishment: Used a research project to identify areas of risk; identified resource allocation issues as a foundation for patient safety.

The Organization

Access Community Health Network (ACCESS) has grown into a large multisite primary care practice organization during its 17-year history. ACCESS provides both primary and specialty health care services in 330 Federally Qualified Health Centers (FQHCs) located in 23 of Chicago's 77 community areas and 11 suburban locations. This extensive network works to fulfill its mission *to provide high-quality, comprehensive community-based health care for the underserved in the greater Chicago area.* Each of the FQHCs requires governance by a patient-majority board of directors with cultural and geographical representation proportional to its service area. During the past three years, ACCESS provided care to almost 200,000 unique patients and had about 650,000 patient visits. ACCESS employs board-certified and board-eligible physicians and midlevel providers in more than 150 full-time equivalent (FTE) positions. In addition, ACCESS contracts for the services of approximately 125 additional medical providers, including specialists and subspecialists. There are also more than 400 allied health staff, including R.N.s, licensed clinical social workers, medical assistants, health educators, case managers, and outreach workers who provide medical care throughout ACCESS's health center–based primary and preventive care network. An additional 150 administrative staff provide support at all of the sites.

ACCESS offers a comprehensive range of medical care and supportive services through its network of community health centers, including primary care, obstetrics and gynecology, substance abuse screening and linkage to treatment, mental health treatment, case management, benefits counseling, and other enabling services to promote patient health. ACCESS supplements primary care services with a variety of specialty services, such as allergy/immunology, cardiology, infectious disease, podiatry, psychiatry, and gastroenterology. Additional services target specific high-risk populations, including immigration physical examinations given at multiple sites, a health center serving developmentally disabled adults, and another serving as a practice center for the three-year family medicine residency.

Project Beginnings
Project Name and Goals
The Risk Assessment of The Testing System (RATTS). Project Goals were to do the following:

1. Gather evidence to identify the steps where errors are most likely to occur in managing laboratory and imaging tests within primary care practices (specifically community health centers).
2. Share the information with clinical staff and obtain feedback.
3. Develop a plan for improving the testing process and present to leadership.

Needs Identification and Baseline Measures

The purpose of this initiative was to comprehensively study the laboratory testing process as a system. The initiative was not designed to examine the performance of any specific individuals within the health center nor specific roles within the testing process. The focus was not on whether tests ordered were clinically indicated or accurately interpreted. Instead, testing was studied as an office system or process. This initiative offered the organization an excellent way to introduce and demonstrate the value of quality improvement research and the potential of research to contribute to patient safety.

Case Study: The Testing Process (continued)

Team Members and Roles

The project team consisted of Milton "Mickey" Eder, Ph.D., Director of Research Programs for the multisite primary care practice; a research assistant at 0.5 FTE and a research assistant (Julia Shklovskaya) already working in the organization; the director of Quality Improvement (Jeni Fabian) also contributed. Three academic researchers contributed significantly to all facets of this project: John Hickner, M.D.; Nancy Elder, M.D.; and Sandy Smith, Ph.D. The project also benefitted from a medical student summer internship. In addition, a consultant (Glenn Seils) wrote a report on each participating site based on observations and a summary report. Clinical and operations leaders from each site involved in the project voluntarily agreed to participate and were provided individualized reports.

Project Activity

Project Steps

The study proposal was developed with organizational input and approval. It was also judged to be of scientific merit through independent review and was funded in part by the Agency for Healthcare Research and Quality (AHRQ). The study consisted of six major components:

1. Office systems engineering analysis of the testing process by direct observation and key informant interviews
2. Chart audit of testing processes and outcomes
3. Patient phone survey
4. Assessment of the management of critical abnormal test results of four tests (Pap smears, mammograms, international normalized ratios [INRs, for coagulation measurement], and prostate-specific antigens)
5. Event reporting
6. A medical office safety culture survey

The team choose 10 representative health centers to study, believing that the lessons learned could be applied to the other 30 health centers.

Adaptation of Existing Hospital Resources

An existing simple event reporting form used in prior primary care safety studies was used to collect event report data. The AHRQ of the Medical Office Safety Culture Survey (http://www.ahrq.gov/qual/mosurvey08/medoffsurv.htm) was used to assess the culture of safety. Questions were added about the testing process and to differentiate views of clinicians and support staff.

For example, the team split the survey query, "(D.7) Staff feel like their mistakes are held against them," into two separate queries: 1. Providers feel . . . and 2. Staff feel . . . . Responses from the different cohorts were very different and shed light on patient safety and just culture issues such as willingness to discuss errors, mistakes, problems, and near misses. In addition, it also suggests that a lack of perceived openness on the part of practices for input from all staff may need to be addressed to develop a strong foundation for successful practice improvement activities.

The Tools Used

The tools used are presented here as well as online as extra material. The two tools included here are Figure 2-3 (chart audit form), page 28, and Figure 2-4 (audit form for critical abnormal labs), page 29. Also used were a testing practice survey, a patient phone survey script and data collection tools, and consent forms. These were all available in both English and Spanish.

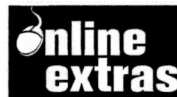

online extras To view additional tools used in this case study, visit the Online Extras at http://www.jcrinc.com/PSAC09/extras/.

Old Process/Plan vs. New

The testing process demonstrated variation both within and between sites. A major source of variation involved the organization of logs used to maintain specimen and referral tracking and logs used for abnormal test/imaging follow-up. Variation existed in staff knowledge about the testing process and the extent of staff responsibilities. Variation was in part the result of site size and number of staff, number and

(continued on page 28)

Case Study: The Testing Process (continued)

Figure 2-3. Testing Process Chart Audit Data Form

Routine Lab Test Audit Form   Date of Audit: _____/_____/_____

Directions:
- This form can be used to assess how well your office documents the lab testing process.
  - ☐ Marking responses on the right side of the page will allow you to place audits next to one another for comparison.
  - ☐ To complete your assessment, line the audits up so that the "no" columns can be seen on multiple pages. →
  - ☐ Checking the "no" circle multiple times for the same question points to areas for improvement.

- If you include the dates in your audit, you can also assess the amount of time it takes to complete different phases of the testing process by reading down the column of dates.

- You can sort your audits according to race/ethnicity to check if the management of patients within the testing process is consistent.

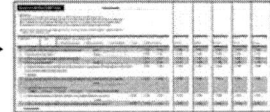

Patient I.D.	DOB	Race/Ethnicity (check all that apply)					
		⃝ Black/African-Amer	⃝ White/Caucasian	⃝ Latino/Hispanic	⃝ Asian	⃝ Native American	⃝ unknown

1. Is there an order for this test in the patient chart?   (Date: ____/____/_____)   ⃝ Yes   ⃝ No

2. Is the test result in the chart?   (Date: ____/____/_____)   ⃝ Yes   ⃝ No

3. Is there a provider signature on the test result?   ⃝ Yes   ⃝ No

   Is this signature dated?   (Date: ____/____/_____)   ⃝ Yes   ⃝ No

4. Is there evidence in the chart of the provider's response to the test result?   ⃝ Yes   ⃝ No

   (e.g. normal, needs further test, etc.)

   Comment:

5. Is there documentation in the chart that the patient was notified of the test results?   ⃝ Yes   ⃝ No

   (Date: ____/____/_____)

   If yes, how was the patient notified?   ⃝ Mail   ⃝ Phone   ⃝ E-mail   ⃝ Pt called   ⃝ No method documented

6. Is there documentation that the patient was notified of follow-up plans?   ⃝ N/A   ⃝ Yes   ⃝ No

   (Date: ____/____/_____)

7. Is there documentation that the patient acknowledged follow-up plans?   ⃝ N/A   ⃝ Yes   ⃝ No

   Comments:

This project was supported by grant number R18HS017911-01 from the Agency for Healthcare Research and Quality.

Initial assessment of processes was achieved with this chart audit form.

Source: Access Community Health Network. Tool developed and provided by John Hickner, M.D., Nancy Elder, M.D., Sandy Smith Ph.D., Mickey Eder, Ph.D., and Eric Chen (MSII).

type of clinicians, and patient insurance or lack thereof, which impacts the number of external labs used. The availability of imaging or mammography services also impacted the number of external relationships to be managed and from which consult reports might originate. Some variation is unavoidable.

The organization was concerned with HIPAA compliance, considering it works with underserved and low socioeconomic minority populations who frequent change housing and have irregular and uncertain phone service. This resulted in policies that did not support communicating protected health information by mail or phone.

Recommended changes were to do the following:
1. Develop policy for informing all patients of both normal and abnormal results.
2. Develop a consistent audit trail and system for maintaining logs for all samples, test results, and follow-up.
3. Verify that patients kept follow-up appointments for abnormal results and contact immediately when

Case Study: The Testing Process (continued)

Figure 2-4. Audit Form for Critical Abnormal Labs

Critical Abnormal Lab Test Audit Form Date of Audit: _____/_____/_____

Directions:

- This form can be used to assess how well your office documents follow-up for critical abnormal lab tests.
  - ☐ Marking responses on the right side of the page will allow you to place audits next to one another for comparison.
  - ☐ To complete your assessment, line the audits up so that the "no" columns can be seen on multiple pages. ➡
  - ☐ Checking the "no" circle multiple times for the same question points to areas for improvement.
- You can sort your audits according to race/ethnicity to check if the management of patients within the testing process is consistent.

Patient I.D.	DOB	Race/Ethnicity (check all that apply)
		○ Black/African-Amer ○ White/Caucasian ○ Latino/Hispanic ○ Asian ○ Native American ○ unknown

1. Is there an order for this test in the patient chart?	○ Yes	○ No
2. Is the test result in the chart?	○ Yes	○ No
3. Is there a provider signature on the test result?	○ Yes	○ No
Is this signature dated?	○ Yes	○ No
4. Is there evidence (documentation) of the provider's response to the test result in the chart? (e.g. normal, needs further test, etc.)	○ Yes	○ No
Comment:		
5. Is there documentation in the chart that the patient was notified of the test result?	○ Yes	○ No
If yes, how was the patient notified? ○ Mail ○ Phone ○ E-mail ○ Pt called ○ No method documented		
6. Is there documentation that the patient was notified of follow-up plans?	○ Yes	○ No
7. Is there documentation that the patient acknowledged follow-up plans?	○ Yes	○ No

Mark which test is being audited and then answer the corresponding questions.

Test	Critical Abnormal Lab Criteria	Questions		
○ Pap Smear	low-grade or high-grade (LGSIL) (HGSIL)	Was the patient notified of the abnormal result within 2 weeks?	○ Yes	○ No
		Did the patient receive follow-up care within 3 months?	○ Yes	○ No
○ Mammogram	BIRAD score of zero or 3 or greater on the report	Was the patient notified of the abnormal result within 2 weeks?	○ Yes	○ No
		Did the patient receive follow-up care within 3 months?	○ Yes	○ No
○ INR Value	INR less than 1.5 or greater than 4.5 in patient on coumadin	Was the patient notified of the abnormal result within 24 hours?	○ Yes	○ No
		Did the patient receive instructions about what to do within 24 hours?	○ Yes	○ No
○ PSA	Values ≥ 4.0	Was the patient notified of the abnormal result within 2 weeks?	○ Yes	○ No
		Did the patient receive follow-up care within 3 months?	○ Yes	○ No
○ other		Was the patient notified of the abnormal result within an appropriate time?	○ Yes	○ No
		Did the patient receive follow-up care within an appropriate time?	○ Yes	○ No

Comments:

This project was supported by grant number R18HS017911-01 from the Agency for Healthcare Research and Quality.

Critical abnormal lab results were assessed using this form. BI-RAD, breast imaging reporting and data system; HGSIL, high-grade squamous intraepithelial lesion; INR, international normalized ratio; LGSIL, low-grade squamous intraepithelial lesion; PSA, prostate-specific antigen; SIL, squamous intraepithelial lesions (on Pap smear).

Source: Access Community Health Network. Tool developed and provided by John Hickner, M.D., Nancy Elder, M.D., Sandy Smith Ph.D., Mickey Eder, Ph.D., and Eric Chen (MSII).

appointment is missed.

4. Regularly review all logs on at least a weekly basis.

5. Determine best practices. Putting results directly into medical records prior to putting results in mail slots increases the risk of losing an abnormal result.

6. Provide medical assistants with dedicated time to keep the logs up to date.

7. Redesign waived testing lab form to include clinician signature.

8. Require labs to inform the health center by start of next business day if test is canceled.

9. Experiment with documenting that patient understood required follow-up on abnormal lab results and potential impact on health outcomes.

Staff Training and Education

Reports combining individual health center data in comparison to aggregate data were provided to all

(continued on page 30)

Case Study: The Testing Process (continued)

10 participating health centers. Health center staff identified areas for improvement based on site-specific performance. To improve particular aspects of the testing process, staff members have begun to develop and implement targeted changes that they developed following review of the individualized report. Health center staff are being supported by the research office to monitor the results of changes to the system.

A report based on the medical office safety culture survey was made to the patient safety committee. This report concerned staff perceptions of safety and quality and processes for improving methods of reporting on mistakes and responses to staff error reports. A report combining all data sources was made to ACCESS leadership with recommendations for improving the testing process within the health centers.

A slide presentation reviewing research results was made to the All Providers' Meeting. More than 120 clinicians were in attendance at this quarterly meeting. The presentation emphasized an awareness of office system integration and the need to monitor systems to curtail variation within systems or processes, particularly the amount of dedicated staff time necessary to adequately manage the laboratory testing process. Informal discussions occurred throughout the data collection and reporting phases with health center staff, clinicians, and organizational leaders.

The Outcome
Measurable Outcomes
Outcomes from the risk assessment study provided evidence for areas of high risk. These areas include the communication between health centers and labs, reporting results to patients, and monitoring patients through follow-up on abnormal labs. Communication breakdowns in reporting and acting on results can directly impact patient health outcomes.

Lessons Learned
Staff embraced almost all aspects of this initiative and responded to reporting results in tremendously

positive ways. The biggest obstacle for improvement continues to be balancing two divergent strategic responses to what was learned. On the one hand, the recommendations could be the basis for a policy that would be developed and instituted in a top-down approach. This approach would have the organization institute new policies to rectify problems that were discovered. On the other hand, considering the variation and unique issues of the participating sites, it would also be possible to develop small-scale initiatives that target problems identified by the staff as the basis for quality improvement. This approach would require more resources, but it would allow individual sites to develop practice and quality improvement skills. Given the dearth of research in this area, the research team did not presume to have genuinely identified best practices. By providing opportunities to test different strategies for improving the testing process, the approach could lead to the development or identification of best practices, while facilitating health center staff education and engagement in quality improvement activities.

One major obstacle involves the safety culture of the organization. The willingness of staff to identify and discuss mistakes involves a level of trust that the medical office safety culture survey indicates is not uniformly present. It is important to explain the goals of the initiative to all staff and to provide opportunities for staff from various sites to talk about the practice improvement activities at their site.

At least one important recommendation involves a change in organizational policy and a commitment to instituting a just culture. Changing policies takes time and in the interim may give the false impression that the issue is not important or that nothing is being done.

Another obstacle involves the impending implementation of an electronic health record (EHR) and staff's unrealistic expectation that this will resolve all the tracking and communication issues and problems. The team has not yet identified how they will counter

Case Study: The Testing Process (continued)

this because the implementation of the EHR has not yet begun. In the interim, they continue to encourage improvements targeting patient safety.

Communicating test results and monitoring follow-up require patient cooperation, which clinical staff do not feel sufficiently empowered to effect. Again, this is an aspect of the project that the team is continuing to work on.

This initiative emphasized process or system improvement. The single most critical issue was getting staff to realize that they needed to understand the entire process and that success was dependent on how each staff member fulfilled his or her responsibility.

Subsequent to the risk assessment project, the team received AHRQ support to develop a toolkit for improving the testing process in primary care practices. Many of the toolkit tools will be simplified versions of materials used by the research team. The intention is to provide tools that will allow practice staff—typically too busy and lacking practice improvement and/or research expertise—to collect data easily and efficiently and to organize that data to identify areas for potential improvement.

Chapter 3

MEDICATION USE

A dverse drug-related events account for an estimated 17 million emergency department visits annually in the United States.[1] It is also estimated that 1 in 9 emergency department visits are due to drug-related adverse events, a potentially preventable problem.[1]

The National Coordinating Council for Medication Error Reporting and Prevention, an independent body of 24 national organizations, defines a medication error as "any preventable event that may cause or lead to inappropriate medication use or patient harm while the medication is in the control of the health care professional, patient, or consumer. Such events may be related to professional practice, health care products, procedures, and systems, including prescribing; order communication; product labeling, packaging, and nomenclature; compounding; dispensing; distribution; administration; education; monitoring; and use."[2]

For ambulatory health care (AHC), organizations should focus on a few particular areas, including high-alert medications (insulin and anticoagulants; that is, warfarin, heparin), contrast imaging agents, injection safety and multiuse medication vials, labeling of medications and containers, look-alike/sound-alike (LASA) medications, medication reconciliation (modified for ambulatory settings), safe prescription writing, and safe use of sample medications. A discussion of anesthesia safety is presented in Chapter 4.

High-Alert Medications

If used in error, high-alert (or high-risk) medications bear an increased risk for causing significant harm to patients. The potential to commit mistakes or errors with these drugs is no higher than with other drugs, but the consequences can be greater. Errors occur most often with incorrect dilutions or concentrations, when one of these drugs is transferred to an unlabeled vial, or when indications for drug use or drug administration procedures are misinterpreted.[3]

Table 3-1. General Risk Reduction Strategies for Using High-Alert Medications

- Standardize preparations of all diluted solutions. These solutions should be prepared prior to surgery so they are in ready-to-use or ready-to-administer containers that allow for sterile delivery of a container's contents.
- Do not dilute medications on the surgical field. Although organizations should refrain from using nonstandardized dilutions, a necessary dilution should be performed only by a registered pharmacist. If a medication must be diluted in the operating room (OR), diluting instructions should be precalculated by a pharmacist and readily available for clinical use.
- Use only premixed solutions and limit the number of medication concentrations.
- Have clinicians in the OR communicate verbally all doses of all medications to be administered and clarify the maximum dose with the anesthesia care provider and surgeon.
- Educate nurses, clinical staff, and unlicensed personnel about safely handling and administering high-alert medications.
- Assess and validate clinical competency with handling and administering medications.

Source: The Joint Commission: *Safety in the Operating Room.* Oakbrook Terrace, IL: Joint Commission Resources, 2006.

When using high-alert medications, incorporate risk reduction strategies such as the ones shown in Table 3-1, above.

In ambulatory settings, a few specific issues associated with high-alert drugs deserve special attention. These include using imaging contrast agents, anticoagulants, insulin, and administering chemotherapeutic agents.

Contrast Agents

In ambulatory settings, patient allergies and contrast-induced nephropathy pose significant safety concerns.

Allergies. Physicians often request radiographic studies that use intravascular radiographic contrast media in the course of evaluating a wide spectrum of diseases. Examples include infusion pyelography, computed tomography, and venography. In many cases a radiologist may not be present to supervise these types of studies.

Primary care physicians may be called on to respond to patients with acute adverse reactions to the contrast medium. Because patients undergoing such studies often have coexisting diseases that increase the risk of adverse reaction to contrast media, ambulatory health care providers must anticipate and be ready to treat deteriorating kidney function. Advising patients about the risks of administration should precede any radiographic procedure, and contrast agents must be properly selected. One way to safeguard against allergies is to give patients or accompanying parents or guardians a questionnaire to complete before any contrast-enhanced imaging is performed.

Dillman et al., at the University of Michigan Health System, used the questionnaire presented in Figure 3-1, page 35, in their study evaluating the incidence and severity of acute allergic-like reactions related to IV administration of low-osmolality nonionic iodinated contrast material in pediatric patients.[4] The questionnaire includes questions about allergy history, including previous contrast reactions, other allergies, and asthma.

By using such a questionnaire—as well as, if available, the electronic medical record, radiology information system, or review of reports from previous contrast-enhanced imaging examinations—providers are able to identify factors that might indicate the use of prophylactic premedication to reduce the risk of acute allergic-like reactions in patients at risk. These decisions should be discussed, and guidelines on the subject should be clearly identified. Guidelines should consider when a patient's medical history includes any of the following[4]:

■ Previous allergic-like reactions to iodinated contrast material
■ Multiple (usually four or more) allergies or a severe allergy to another substance (*see* Chapter 4, "Surgical Safety," for more information on this topic)
■ Asthma with frequent, recent, or severe attacks

Legal issues surrounding the selection of radiographic contrast media have surfaced in the courts and state legislative bodies. Numerous local and national organization guidelines exist to guide the physician in appropriately selecting radiographic contrast media, but there is still wide variation in the use of low-osmolarity contrast media by individual physicians, institutions, and geographic location.

Contrast-induced nephropathy. Contrast-induced nephropathy is most commonly defined as acute renal failure occurring within 48 hours after exposure to intravascular radiographic contrast material, not attributable to other causes, and persisting for two to five days.[5] With the increasing use of iodinated contrast media in diagnostic imaging and interventional procedures, particularly for high-risk patients, contrast-induced nephropathy has become a significant source of morbidity and mortality.

The Pennsylvania Patient Safety Authority developed an algorithm tool for examining contrast-related procedures. The tool is duplicated here in Figure 3-2, page 36.

Anticoagulants

Joint Commission requirements call for taking action to reduce the risk of harm associated with the use of anticoagulant therapy.

Anticoagulants are one of the top five drug categories associated with patient safety incidents. Anticoagulants are listed as high-alert medications by the Institute for Safe Medication Practices because of the significant risk of life-threatening bleeding or thrombosis if the appropriate safe practices are not in place. Protocols, guidelines, and standing orders for warfarin and other anticoagulants should be complete and appropriate. Thorough patient education is also important for patients on these drugs (*see* "Patient Education" on pages 7–11 in Chapter 1).

The National Quality Forum (NQF), in its Safety Objective #29, states that "Every patient on long-term oral anticoagulants should be monitored by a qualified health professional using a careful strategy to ensure an appropriate intensity of supervision." The NQF outlines explicit organizational policies and procedures necessary for effectively managing patients taking

Figure 3-1. Questionnaire for Determining Allergy in Pediatric Patients

DEPARTMENT OF RADIOLOGY
CONTRAST REACTION REPORT FORM

PEDIATRIC ONLY

GENERAL INFORMATION

ID NO: _____

Date/Time of Incident: Date _____ Time _____

Inpatient _____ Outpatient _____

Previous Incident: Date _____ Type _____

Date/Time Notified Radiology House Officer _____ Attending Radiologist _____

Attending Physician _____ House Physician _____

DESCRIPTION OF INCIDENT

Contrast Agent Administered _____ Dose _____ Route _____ Length of Time _____

Procedure Done _____

Patient's Normal Blood Pressure _____ Patient's Normal Pulse _____

Patient's Blood Pressure During Incident _____ Patient's Pulse During Incident _____

Pre-Medication Given _____

SYMPTOMS AND SIGNS OF REACTION

CARDIOVASCULAR:

RESPIRATORY:

NERVOUS:

SKIN:

GI TRACT:

OTHER: _____

MEDICAL REPORT

TREATMENT ADMINISTERED

None _____ O$_2$ _____ IV _____ Epinephrine _____

Benadryl _____ Atropine _____ Steroids _____ Aminophylline _____

Cardiopulmonary Resuscitation _____ Other _____

Radiologist Findings _____

Name _____ Date _____ Time _____

Q.A.

Was the contrast reaction kit readily available? _____ Yes _____ No

Were the contents of the reaction kit adequate for this incident? _____ Yes _____ No

Was support equipment, e.g., suction equipment, O$_2$, etc., readily available? _____ Yes _____ No

Did you have enough support in the management of this contrast reaction? _____ Yes _____ No

RP-2090341D/S Rev. 10/96	RADIOLOGY		CONTRAST REACTION REPORT

Caregivers of children completed this questionnaire to determine allergies before any procedure was performed. This form can be adapted for use in the ambulatory setting.

Source: Dillman J.R., et al.: Incidence and severity of acute allergic-like reactions to i.v. nonionic iodinated contrast material in children. *Am J Roentgenol* 188:1643–1647, Jun. 2007.

Figure 3-2. Algorithm for the Management of Patients Undergoing Iodinated Contrast-Related Procedures

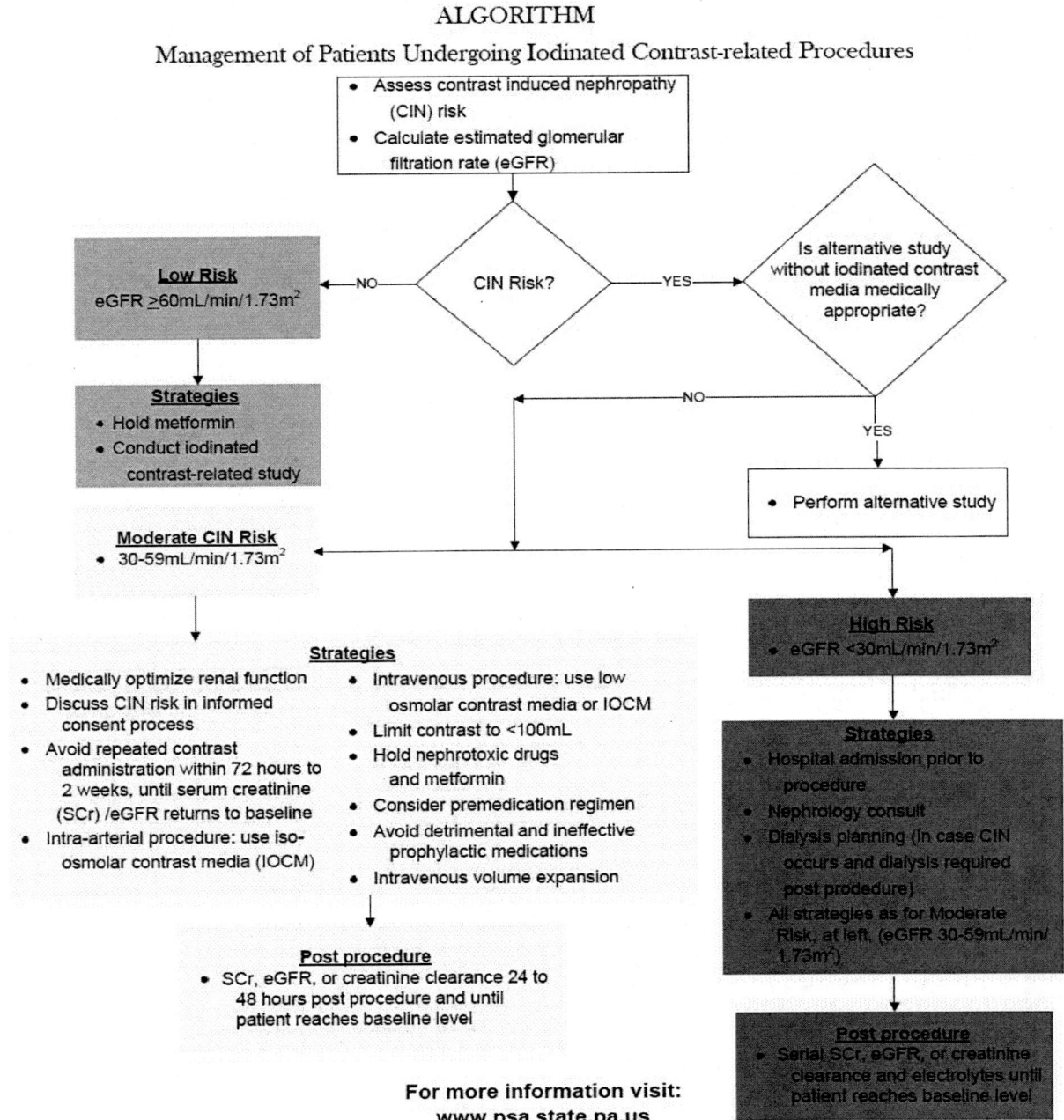

ALGORITHM

Management of Patients Undergoing Iodinated Contrast-related Procedures

- Assess contrast induced nephropathy (CIN) risk
- Calculate estimated glomerular filtration rate (eGFR)

CIN Risk?

NO → **Low Risk** eGFR $\geq$60mL/min/1.73m^2

YES → **Is alternative study without iodinated contrast media medically appropriate?**

NO →

YES → **Perform alternative study**

Low Risk Strategies:
- Hold metformin
- Conduct iodinated contrast-related study

Moderate CIN Risk
- 30-59mL/min/1.73m^2

High Risk
- eGFR <30mL/min/1.73m^2

Strategies (Moderate)
- Medically optimize renal function
- Discuss CIN risk in informed consent process
- Avoid repeated contrast administration within 72 hours to 2 weeks, until serum creatinine (SCr) /eGFR returns to baseline
- Intra-arterial procedure: use iso-osmolar contrast media (IOCM)
- Intravenous procedure: use low osmolar contrast media or IOCM
- Limit contrast to <100mL
- Hold nephrotoxic drugs and metformin
- Consider premedication regimen
- Avoid detrimental and ineffective prophylactic medications
- Intravenous volume expansion

Strategies (High)
- Hospital admission prior to procedure
- Nephrology consult
- Dialysis planning (in case CIN occurs and dialysis required post procedure)
- All strategies as for Moderate Risk, at left, (eGFR 30-59mL/min/1.73m^2)

Post procedure (Moderate)
- SCr, eGFR, or creatinine clearance 24 to 48 hours post procedure and until patient reaches baseline level

Post procedure (High)
- Serial SCr, eGFR, or creatinine clearance and electrolytes until patient reaches baseline level

For more information visit:
www.psa.state.pa.us

This algorithm was adapted from "Contrast-Induced Nephropathy: Can This Iatrogenic Complication of Iodinated Contrast be Prevented?" *PA-PSRS Patient Safety Advisory.* March 30, 2007. Vol. 4, Suppl. 1.

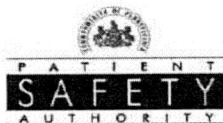

© 2007 Pennsylvania Patient Safety Authority

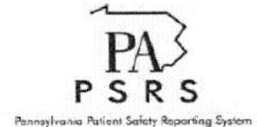

PATIENT SAFETY AUTHORITY

PA PSRS
Pennsylvania Patient Safety Reporting System

This tool can be posted in the diagnostic imaging suite.

Source: ECRI Institute and Institute for Safe Medication Practices: Contrast-induced nephropathy: Can this iatrogenic complication of iodinated contrast be prevented? *PA-PSRS Patient Safety Advisory* 4(suppl. 1), Mar. 30, 2007.

Figure 3-3. Outpatient Anticoagulation Flow Sheet

Patient's Name _____   MRN _____
Phone _____   Physician _____

Indication _____   Duration _____   INR goal _____

Date	PT/INR POC/venous	Current Regimen	New Regimen	Next Lab	MD Notified/Initials

Source: Purdue University PharmaTAP: *Anticoagulation Toolkit: Reducing Adverse Drug Events and Potential Adverse Drug Events with Unfractionated Heparin, Low Molecular Weight Heparins and Warfarin.* 2008. http://www.purdue.edu/dp/rche/about/centers/pharmatap/pdf/toolkit.pdf (accessed Sep. 27, 2009).

Table 3-2. Common Risks and Safe Practices Associated with Anticoagulants

Common Risks	Safe Practices
■ Duplicate or concurrent therapy ■ Accidental stoppage of therapy ■ Look-alike vials or syringes ■ Look-alike names ■ Dosing errors ■ Calculation errors ■ Monitoring problems ■ Food and drug interactions ■ Spinal hematoma ■ Adverse drug reactions ■ Confusion between insulin and heparin; between LMWHs and UFH	■ Avoid reliance on memory by: —Using protocols/checklists —Automating —Developing built-in reminders ■ Simplify tasks by: —Decreasing steps in the process —Decreasing number of staff involved in the process —Reducing need for calculations ■ Reduce or eliminate handoffs. ■ Standardize by developing practice guidelines, order sets, and pathways. ■ Use constraints and forcing functions by: —Ensuring use of required computer fields —Removing outdated forms —Utilizing free-flow pump protection ■ Improve access to information.

Key: LMWH, low molecular weight heparin; UFH, unfractionated heparin.

Source: Adapted from Institute for Safe Medication Practices, *Medication Safety Alert* 12, Jan. 11, 2007.

---

anticoagulants. Using anticoagulants requires careful thinking and attention to detail.[6] Risks and safe practices for anticoagulant use are presented in Table 3-2, above.

Other useful tools to track patients' anticoagulant use is the outpatient flow sheet presented in Figure 3-3, above, and the outpatient warfarin dosing card, presented in Figure 3-4, page 38.

Insulin

Diabetes care is becoming increasingly standardized with the use of disease state management systems.[7] One way that care has improved is that many providers, at the actual point of patient contacts, are using point-of-care testing and employing sliding scales to modify doses of insulin.

Standardization will also be strengthened by the growing use of computerized tools. If your practice site

Figure 3-4. Outpatient Warfarin Dosing Card

ANTICOAGULATION CLINIC _____

_____

Your Warfarin dose has been changed. You should now take:

| 1 mg
Red | 2 mg
Purple | 2.5 mg
Green | 4 mg
Blue | 5 mg
Peach | 6 mg
Blue-Grn | 6.5 mg
Yellow | 10 mg
White |

Number of tablets to take each day:

Strength	Color	Sun	Mon	Tues	Wed	Thur	Fri	Sat

Date: _____ Name: _____

Next Appointment: _____

- -

ANTICOAGULATION CLINIC _____

Wishard Health Services

Number of tablets to take each day:

Strength	Color	Sun	Mon	Tues	Wed	Thur	Fri	Sat

Date: _____ Name: _____

Next Appointment: _____

Source: Purdue University PharmaTAP: *Anticoagulation Toolkit: Reducing Adverse Drug Events and Potential Adverse Drug Events with Unfractionated Heparin, Low Molecular Weight Heparins and Warfarin.* 2008. http://www.purdue.edu/dp/rche/about/centers/pharmatap/pdf/toolkit.pdf (accessed Sep. 27, 2009).

is not yet fully implemented with electronic media for medication order entry, you should standardize paper-based tools and protocols to ensure safe insulin use.

Chemotherapy Administration

Chemotherapy drugs also top the list of high-alert medications.[8] Apply safeguards to chemotherapy administration by standardizing and quality-checking medication preparation and administration; addressing skill mix, competency, and productivity issues; implementing a means to educate staff, addressing questions of both staff and patients; and clearly communicating drug orders. These issues are detailed in the sections below.

Medication preparation and administration. Because chemotherapy is individualized and nonstandardized, preparation of medications is a potential area for risk.[8] Doses are prepared based on body size or other factors,

such as kidney function, and require accurate patient-specific calculations. Sometimes doses must be adjusted, which means additional calculations must be made. Also, most chemotherapy drugs require reconstitution and preparation. Some agents are available in multidose vials and varying concentrations. Another risk is that drugs can be administered subcutaneously or via IV. They are given in differing doses (standard versus high dose) and over varying periods of time (bolus versus continuous infusion).

Skill mix and productivity issue for administrations. Some states require that a registered nurse (R.N.) administer chemotherapy agents. Because complex, multidrug protocols are often used for cancer therapy, there is an increased risk for errors.[8] These tasks cannot be delegated to lesser-qualified staff. This influences staff work schedules and productivity issues. Furthermore, introducing new agents occurs regularly,

Table 3-3. Chemotherapy Error Prevention Principles	
Principle	**Implementation**
Proactive approach	■ Conduct ongoing review of chemotherapy prescription, transcription, preparation, administration, and patient monitoring processes. ■ Make needed procedural changes before an error occurs. ■ Review "near miss" events (close calls).
Multidisciplinary participation	■ Involve everyone who has a role in chemotherapy error prevention (for example, unit secretaries, patient educators, pharmacy couriers who transport chemotherapy, and so on). ■ Promote team identification.
Open communication	■ Empower health care providers to "speak up" and share ideas and safety concerns. ■ Encourage patients to ask questions and express concerns.
Systems analysis	■ Examine the overall system of chemotherapy administration and identify how one component can potentially affect another (a flowchart may be helpful to illustrate this process). ■ Conduct a Failure Mode and Effects Analysis (FMEA), which focuses on three aspects of a process (likelihood of failure, chances of failure causing harm, and the likelihood of the failure being undetected).
Redesign vulnerable patient systems	■ Use human factors engineering to identify and correct system failures (for example, processes, equipment, and so on). (*See* Chapter 7, "Staff Education and Training.")
Safe practice	■ Provide evidence-based care. ■ Adhere to institutional policies and procedures. ■ Review and revise procedures periodically (at least annually). ■ Update and revise procedures as new information becomes available.
Information transfer	■ Review how information is recorded, relayed, and stored. ■ Use information technology (for example, electronic medical records, personal digital assistants such as handhelds and smartphones, and so on).
Education, competency, and credentialing	■ Evaluate prospective and current employees' educational preparation, experience, and present knowledge and skill level. ■ Identify and address deficiencies. ■ Provide and support continuing education. ■ Encourage and support board and specialty certification. ■ Delineate credentialing criteria (for example, specify who has the authority to prescribe and administer chemotherapy).
Culture of safety	■ Emphasize safety and error prevention. ■ Create patient safety specialist positions or teams. ■ Demonstrate leadership's support for safety initiatives. (Safety needs to be a priority from the top down.) ■ Create a nonpunitive environment for expressing safety concerns and reporting errors. ■ Consider related areas that impact safety, such as safely handling chemotherapy. ■ Avoid "naming, blaming, and shaming" individuals involved in chemotherapy errors and instead ask, "How did this happen?"
Continuous quality improvement	■ Ensure that error prevention is a continuous process that includes ongoing informal evaluation and a more formal evaluation on a periodic basis. ■ Use prospective methods to prevent chemotherapy errors (for example, observational methods).

Source: Schulmeister L.: Preventing chemotherapy errors. *Oncologist* 11:463–468, May 2006.

Table 3-4. Error Prevention Recommendations for Chemotherapy Prescribing and Preparation

Chemotherapy Orders

- Develop a list of required elements, including patient data, that each set of chemotherapy orders must contain.
- Use standardized preprinted order forms or computerized prescriber order entry systems with built-in approved protocols and alerts.
- Never give verbal orders for chemotherapy.
- Use a high-quality fax machine to receive chemotherapy orders and avoid faxing "copies of copies."
- Handwrite chemotherapy orders in printed block letters or enter electronically.
- Write, imprint, or enter the patient's full name on chemotherapy order forms.
- Write or enter the date and time the chemotherapy orders are generated, and state the date and time chemotherapy is to be administered if different from the order date and time. Use military time, print "AM" and "PM" or use another identifier, such as "12 noon" to avoid confusion.
- Review the patient's allergy and drug-related adverse event history.
- Calculate or confirm body surface area calculation.
- Review the patient's data (for example, diagnosis and stage of disease, laboratory test results, patient's weight) and select the initial treatment protocol. For subsequent treatments, review patient data to determine if dose escalation or reduction is indicated.
- Review the patient's treatment records. Confirm that an appropriate time interval has elapsed since the patient's last treatment. Determine the patient's cumulative chemotherapy dose when indicated.
- Review the patient's response to treatment and identify treatment-related toxicity that may require dose adjustment or a new treatment plan.
- Specify drug name, dose, route, and rate. For continuous chemotherapy infusions, state daily dose and total dose to be administered.
- Specify sequencing of chemotherapy agents to be administered when applicable.
- Spell out generic names of chemotherapy agents.
- Spell out the word *units*.
- Use a consistent dose form, such as milligrams (mg), for all doses.
- Do not use trailing zeros for any dose ≥ 1 mg (for example, 2 mg).
- Always place a leading zero in doses < 1 mg (for example, 0.8 mg).
- Double-check dose calculations.
- Check to see that chemotherapy orders are complete and include antiemetics, hydration, protective agents, and growth factors when indicated. Order test doses of chemotherapy if applicable. Specify patient monitoring parameters and frequency when indicated.
- Sign the orders and include contact information (for example, phone or pager number) when required.

Chemotherapy Preparation

- Clearly label stock bins of chemotherapy agents. Place "look-alike, sound-alike" alerts on bins containing chemotherapy agents with similarly appearing or sounding names.
- Review the patient's allergy and drug-related adverse event history.
- Review the patient's data (for example, laboratory test results, patient's weight) and treatment protocol to determine if the chemotherapy orders are consistent with the protocol and appropriate for the patient.
- Review the patient's treatment records. Confirm that an appropriate time interval has elapsed since the patient's last treatment. Confirm the patient's cumulative chemotherapy dose if applicable.
- Review the chemotherapy orders. Recalculate chemotherapy doses. Obtain additional information or clarification when indicated.
- Calculate and recheck preparation computations (for example, diluent volumes, final concentrations, additives, overfill, dose) and note special directions, such as using a filter to prepare the drug.
- Prepare labels and include storage and expiration information.
- Select vials of chemotherapy that contain appropriate dose strengths and, when applicable, note the amount that must be discarded to equal the patient's prescribed dose. Examine expiration dates on the vials and record drug lot numbers.
- Recheck chemotherapy preparation calculations.
- Compare prepared labels with chemotherapy orders to ensure that the patient's name, drug, dose, route, and time match.
- Prepare chemotherapy in accordance with manufacturers' recommendations, inspect final solution, and apply labels.
- Place prepared chemotherapy in a plastic bag and have it transported for administration or store the agents according to the manufacturer's recommendations.

Chemotherapy Administration

- Review the patient's allergy and drug-related adverse event history.
- Review the patient's data (for example, laboratory test results, patient's weight) and treatment protocol to confirm that doses are appropriate and correct.
- Review the patient's treatment records. Confirm that an appropriate time interval has elapsed since the patient's last treatment. Confirm the patient's cumulative chemotherapy dose when indicated.
- Review the patient's response to treatment and identify treatment-related toxicity that may require symptom management.

(continued on page 41)

Table 3-4. Error Prevention
Recommendations for Chemotherapy
Prescribing and Preparation (continued)

- Review the chemotherapy orders. Confirm that all required elements are present, including ancillary medications such as antiemetics, and patient monitoring instructions. Recalculate chemotherapy doses. Obtain additional information or clarification when indicated.
- Compare the labels on the prepared chemotherapy agents with the chemotherapy orders and treatment plan or protocol. Note if specific sequencing of agents is prescribed.
- Provide patient teaching verbally or in writing.
- Verify patient identity using two identifiers. Ask patients to state the last four digits of their social security number or their complete address or show their driver's license or other photo identification.
- Administer chemotherapy agents as prescribed.
- Monitor the patient for adverse events, such as hypersensitivity reaction, chemotherapy infiltration, vesicant extravasation, and so on.
- Provide or reinforce postchemotherapy patient teaching, including instructions on self-care, monitoring and reporting side effects, symptom management, and so on.

Source: Adapted from Schulmeister L.: Preventing chemotherapy errors. *Oncologist* 11:463–468, May 2006.

Table 3-5. Risk Reduction Strategies for
Injection Administration and Use of
Multiuse Medication Vials

- Discard single-use ampules and vials after the contents have been drawn up. Discard prefilled syringes after use. A single-dose ampule, vial, or prefilled syringe containing medication intended for single use generally does not contain the bacteriostatic or preservative agents found in multidose vials.
- Draw up the medication as close to administration time as possible to best avoid contamination with bacteria or other microorganisms from nonsterile glass fragments, airborne contaminants, or failure to use aseptic technique.
- Do not use syringes and needles (single-use sterile items) for multiple patients, even if the needle is changed.
- Discard all used needles and syringes into a sharps container.
- Discard multidose vials with suspected or visible contamination, and those that are outdated. Breaks in aseptic technique can introduce microbial contamination into the vial via the needle, syringe, or rubber stopper. (For example, outbreaks of viral and bacterial infections, including hepatitis B, have been traced to contaminated multidose vials.)

Source: Blanchard J.: Environmental controls; multiuse syringes and needles; patient identification; *Staphylococcus aureus*—Clinical Issues—question and answer. *AORN J* Jun. 2003.

and clinical staff must update themselves on the newest knowledge.

Responding to staff and patients' questions. In most chemotherapy clinics, a dedicated pharmacist is generally not available to address questions and educate staff. Some means to address these questions must be provided and be easily accessible.

Communicating orders clearly. In a series of administration cycles, the nurse must keep track of manual orders and which cycle the patient is in. This does not pertain to clinics using automated systems. Put systems in place for clear communication regarding ordering, preparing, dispensing, and administering chemotherapy. Communication will involve many parts of an organization, each juncture of transitions (handoffs), and people from differing backgrounds and experience. Communication is also at risk when information technology and software are not integrated.

It is important to use these safe practices for

chemotherapy ordering, preparation, and administration. Table 3-3, page 39, presents prevention principles and techniques found useful in ambulatory chemotherapy clinics. The National Coordinating Council on Medication Error Reporting and Prevention also emphasizes that verbal orders should never be used with antineoplastic agents (*see* http://www.nccmerp.org/council/council2001-02-20. html). Additional error prevention strategies are shown in Table 3-4, pages 40–41.

Injection Safety and Multiuse Medication Vials

In January 2008, investigators from the Centers for Disease Control and Prevention's (CDC's) Division of Viral Hepatitis and Division of Healthcare Quality Promotion investigated a report in Nevada that three persons with acute hepatitis C virus had undergone procedures at a Las Vegas endoscopy clinic. Ultimately, a total of six cases of hepatitis C infection were identified. On investigation, the CDC and the Southern Nevada Health District determined that practices that had the potential to transmit hepatitis C were used at the facility.[9,10]

Unsafe injection practices—primarily reusing syringes and needles or contaminating multiple-dose medication vials—has led to patient-to-patient transmission in a private physician practice in New York, a pain remediation clinic in Oklahoma, and a hematology-oncology clinic in Nebraska.[11] As of fall 2008, other investigations were in progress in Michigan and North Carolina. The root causes underlying these outbreaks appear to be multifactorial, rooted in a combination of events, and include a lack of understanding and adherence to the most basic safe injection practice (that is, reusing single-use syringes, biopsy forceps, and medication [propofol] vials) and a recognized lack of adequate comprehensive systems for professional training and oversight of infection control protocols[12] (see Chapter 5, "Infection Prevention and Control").

In their "Recommendations for Infection Control for the Practice of Anesthesiology," the American Society of Anesthesiologists states that they support the practice of using aseptic technique, using multiuse vials appropriately, and not reusing syringes and needles.[13] A number of factors can affect whether medications become contaminated and lead to the growth of organisms. Strategies for injection safety and use of multiuse vials are presented in Table 3-5, page 41.

It is important to note that Standard MM.03.01.01, EP 10, requires that all stored medications be labeled with the expiration date (defined as the last date that the product should be used—also called the "beyond use" date). All current standards of practice related to expiration dating of multidose vials (such as from the Association for Professionals in Infection Control and Epidemiology, United States Pharmacopeia, and Centers for Medicare & Medicaid Services) require that multidose vials be discarded 28 days after opening, or by the manufacturer's expiration date, whichever is less. After a multidose vial is opened, the revised expiration date (28 days later) should be put on the label, and the product discarded after that time or sooner, if the manufacturer date is sooner.

Labeling Medications and Containers

Joint Commission requirements call for labeling all medications, medication containers (for example, syringes, medicine cups, basins), or other solutions on and off the sterile field.

In the AHC setting, certain activities and processes can be undertaken to improve labeling risks. Do not base medication selection solely on label color-coding. Color-coding has been associated with selection errors, and similar problems occur when labels are molded into medication packaging such as plastic ampoules, or are devoid of color. A wise approach to accurate medication selection is to check the medication package and label during selection and before administration. Also, have a coworker review the selected agent for accuracy in name, dose, strength, and expiration date.[14]

Patients' misunderstanding of instructions on prescription drug labels is common and also contributes to medication errors and reduced treatment effectiveness.[15] Using precise wording on prescription drug label instructions has been shown to improve patient comprehension. However, patients with limited literacy are more likely to misinterpret instructions. (See Chapter 1, "Patient-Centered Care," for strategies to help patients reduce the risk of errors with medications used outside the health care setting.)

Labeling confusion of medications plays a role in as many as half of all medication errors.[16] Labels may be printed in small type, have similar designs and layouts, or have similar colors, designs, or type. In addition, labels may be confused when placed on vials that are similar in size or shape.

Problems with labeling, as well as with similar looking or sounding medication names (see the section beginning on page 43 of this chapter), are not the only issues involved in these types of medication errors. Other contributing factors include the following[16]:

- Poor handwriting, particularly faint or illegible script
- Abbreviation of medication names
- Protocols such as chemotherapy are written in acronyms (for example, CHOP, ABVD)
- Referring to medications by nicknames (for example, "Donna" for daunorubicin, "epi" for epirubicin)
- Excessive use of verbal orders, which may be misinterpreted or misunderstood

■ Prescribers placing an incorrect prefix or suffix on the name of a medication, thus creating a word resembling the name of another, unintended medication

■ The introduction of many new medications every year, each with a generic and trade name that may be similar to other drugs already on the market

It is not enough to caution providers to be more careful labeling or accessing vials and containers. It is human nature to identify items by color, shape, typeface, symbols employed, and other such characteristics. To help minimize errors related to nomenclature, labeling, and packaging, consider using the strategy tool presented in Sidebar 3-1, on this page.

A case study concerning medication labeling is presented in this chapter beginning on page 51.

Look-Alike/Sound-Alike Medications

As mentioned previously, many medications have generic or trade names that can look or sound similar. These LASA medication names can increase the risk of unintended interchanges or medication mix-ups leading to harmful errors.

Confirmation bias can play a part in LASA–related errors. Confirmation bias is when a person notices what he or she expects to notice rather than what is really there. In such a case, one ignores evidence that does not confirm one's beliefs or expectations.

The following sentence illustrates an example of confirmation bias: It deosn't mtater how wrods are rwitten bcuseae the huamn mnid deos not raed ervey lteter by istlef, but the wrod as a wlohe.[16] Because human beings often see what they want to see, systems must be made to accommodate this inclination in order to prevent error.

One of the National Patient Safety Goals is to identify annually (at a minimum) a list of LASA drugs used in the organization. Actions must be taken to prevent errors involving the interchange of drugs.[16]

✓ Joint Commission requirements call for organizations to identify and review annually their list of look-alike/sound-alike medications used and determine methods to prevent associated errors.

Sidebar 3-1. Risk Reduction Strategies for Labeling and Containers

■ **Perform a failure mode and effects analysis (FMEA).** Before adding a medication to your organization's inventory, consider gathering an appropriate interdisciplinary team to perform a FMEA to determine potential pitfalls with that medication. Include an evaluation of the look-alike potential of product containers as well as possible areas of storage throughout the organization. This will help identify any necessary steps that must be taken to reduce the risk of errors.

■ **Review reports from external sources.** Regularly review professional literature to identify error-prone drug products.

■ **Purchase from different vendors.** Consider purchasing one product of an identified look-alike pair from a different vendor. This might help reduce similarities and thwart the possibility of errors.

■ **Segregate and label.** Consider separating and clearly differentiating products that are similar, or for extra security, do both.

■ **Establish a system of alerts.** Build alerts into your computer systems to help remind practitioners that certain product issues are problematic.

■ **Use drug-dose conversion charts.** Not all health care practitioners are familiar with percent or ratio expressions of concentrations or adept at calculating the drug doses whose concentrations are expressed this way. Consider consulting drug-dose conversion charts to create a version that solely represents the concentrations available in your facility. Post the chart on code carts and in other areas where emergency medications are prepared. Keep charts useful and up to date by implementing a process for ensuring that they undergo an approval process prior to use. This will help ensure that updates are performed as new products are published.

■ **Document contributing factors.** If you submit reports to a local medication error agency, you may have access to a computerized capability to track contributing factors to adverse events. Such factors might include dosage-form confusion, look-alike and sound-alike issues, or confusing label design. Identifying these products and analyzing the contributing factors can assist quality improvement programs and guide the development of further error prevention strategies.

Source: ECRI Institute and Institute for Safe Medication Practices: Drug labeling and packaging—Looking beyond what meets the eye. *PA-PSRS Patient Safety Advisory* 4:69, 73–77, Sep. 2007.

In an AHC setting, there may be a limited medication stock specific to the population served and the services provided. In such cases, it is important to coordinate with a pharmacist when possible, particularly when questions arise.

TOOL: Visual Controls

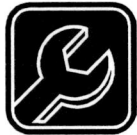

This approach to the design of systems and processes includes the use of any display, card, or visual signal that will help improve clarity and communication, reduce searching times, and reduce safety risks.

You can distinguish and differentiate LASA drugs by applying a system of visual controls. Ideas for such a system are presented in Sidebar 3-2 on this page. A list of problematic medication names used in ambulatory settings are presented in Table 3-6, page 45.

Medication Reconciliation

Joint Commission requirements call for developing a process to compare the patient's current medications with those ordered for the patient while under the care of the organization.

The Institute for Healthcare Improvement defines medication reconciliation as "the process of creating the most accurate list possible of all medications a patient is taking, including drug name, dosage, frequency, and route, and comparing that list against the physician's admission, transfer, and/or discharge orders, with the goal of providing correct medications to the patient at all transition points within a hospital." As of January 2006, The Joint Commission called for having protocols in place for documenting and reconciling medications across the continuum of care.[17]

Given the difficulties that many organizations are having in meeting the complex requirements of the medication reconciliation National Patient Safety Goal, The Joint Commission announced plans in early 2009 for further evaluation and revision of the goal. While this evaluation takes place, the following will occur:

- Surveyors will continue to evaluate compliance with Goal 8 to collect data for Joint Commission process improvement efforts.
- Surveyors' findings will not contribute to an organization's accreditation decision.

> ## Sidebar 3-2. Tips for Look-Alike Sound-Alike (LASA) Use, Dispensing, and Storage
>
> - Do *not* store LASA medications alphabetically by name. Store them out of order or in an alternative location.
> - Limit the stock supply of some medications. (For example, stock only concentrated liquid morphine as opposed to also stocking other morphine concentrations.) Or you might stock an alternative medication without nomenclature issues and eliminate a LASA medication from the formulary.
> - When a new drug is added to the formulary, ask a few clinicians to handwrite the product name and directions as they would in a typical order. These "mock" orders can be given to clinical staff, pharmacists, technicians, or unit secretaries as a trial to read aloud and interpret. New drugs are often mispronounced and that mispronunciation may sound like a medication already in use.
> - Pop-up alerts in interactive computer software can be made visual and auditory. Address with the staff whether overriding alerts is a problem in your organization and what can be done to resolve that habit.
> - Use uppercase (tall man) lettering, italics, and bold type on labels and stock bins (for example, CISplatin, vinCRIStine).
> - Place caution labels on bins containing LASA drugs.
> - Double-, triple-, and quadruple-check all medications on orders. Use different generic and trade names for clarification.
> - Make two independent checks during the medication dispensing process: one person interprets and enters or processes the order, and another compares the printed label against the original order and the medication vial. Change the position of the vial for the first and second check to present a different view that can counter confirmation bias.
>
> Reference: Schulmeister L.: Look-alike, sound-alike oncology medications. *Clin J Oncol Nurs* 10:35-41, Feb. 2006.

- Surveyors' findings will not generate Requirements for Improvement and will not appear on an organization's accreditation report.

Recognizing that medication reconciliation problems put patients at risk, The Joint Commission expects organizations to continue to address medication reconciliation across the continuum of care. Meanwhile, The Joint Commission will create an improved National

Table 3-6. Potentially Problematic Medication Names Used in Ambulatory Settings

For Office-Based Surgery and Ambulatory Surgery Centers

- cisplatin and carboplatin
- doxorubicin liposome and daunorubicin liposome and conventional forms of doxorubicin and daunorubicin
- Taxol (Bristol-Myers Squibb, Princeton, NJ) and Taxotere (Aventis Pharmaceuticals Inc., Bridgewater, NJ)
- vinblastine and vincristine
- lipid-based amphotericin products and conventional forms of amphotericin
- hydromorphone and morphine
- concentrated liquid morphine products and conventional liquid morphine products
- ephedrine and epinephrine
- fentanyl and sulfentanil
- insulin products

For Other Ambulatory Care Settings

- Avandia (GlaxoSmithKline, Research Triangle Park, NC) and Coumadin (Bristol-Myers Squibb)
- Celebrex (Pfizer Inc., New York), Celexa (Forest Pharmaceuticals, Inc., St. Louis), and Cerebyx (Pfizer, Inc.)
- clonidine and Klonopin (Roche Pharmaceuticals, Nutley, NJ)
- Lamisil (Novartis Pharmaceuticals Corp., East Hanover, NJ) and Lamictal (GlaxoSmithKline)
- Serzone (Bristol-Myers Squibb) and Seroquel (AstraZeneca, Wilmington, DE)
- Zyprexa (Eli Lilly and Company, Indianapolis) and Zyrtec (Pfizer, Inc.)
- concentrated liquid morphine products and conventional morphine products
- hydromorphone injection and morphine injection
- insulin products

Source: Schulmeister L.: Look-alike, sound-alike oncology medications. *Clin J Oncol Nurs* 10:35-41, Feb. 2006.

Table 3-7. Medication Reconciliation Assessment Tips

- Ask open-ended questions starting with what, why, and when, and balance them with yes-no questions.
- Ask simple questions and don't use medical jargon. Avoid leading questions that might elicit inaccurate information.
- Prompt patients to recall all medication products they use, including patches, creams, eyedrops or eardrops, inhalers, sample medications, "shots," herbal or mineral supplements, and vitamins.
- Pursue unclear information until it is clarified. For example, check previous medical records, ask a family member to bring in the patient's medications, or call the home pharmacy for a list of prescriptions the patient has been filling.
- Encourage the patient to get all medications from the same pharmacy.
- When questioning patients about adverse events, educate them about the difference between an expected adverse effect and a true allergy and make sure they know which signs and symptoms require immediate attention.
- Ask patients to describe how and when they take their medications, which may help you determine if they are adhering to the prescribed regimen.
- Advise patients to keep a medication wallet card and to bring all medications or a complete list of them to appointments with health care providers or in the event they are hospitalized.

Source: Modified from Manno M.S., Hayes D.D.: How medication reconciliation saves lives *Nursing 36* Mar. 2006. http://www.nursing2006.com/ (accessed Feb.16, 2009).

Patient Safety Goal that both supports quality and safety of care and can be more readily implemented by the health care field in 2010.

An Ambulatory Surgery Foundation survey was conducted to examine the ways ambulatory surgical centers (ASCs) are managing medication reconciliation for their patients.[18] Survey results found a vast number of inconsistencies in what information was collected, the way each ASC collects the information, barriers to compliance, and the way each ASC communicates the information after a procedure. More guidance on implementation is required. The patient's medication list should also include appropriate times and settings for taking a medication, additional pertinent information (such as allergies) and ways to handle temporary changes to the medication list.

Staff should perform medication reconciliation in any setting where medications are used or prescribed. Accurate and complete medication reconciliation can prevent many prescribing and administering errors. The purpose of reconciliation is to avoid errors, including those of transcription, omission, duplication of therapy, and drug-drug and drug-disease interactions. Each organization determines how to make and who will make this comparison. Use clinic databases to list all medications that patients take in the ambulatory setting. Typically, clinical or support staff will update this list with patients prior to their meeting with a physician.[19] (A process map for medication reconciliation appears in Chapter 2 as Figure 2-2 on page 21.) The case study beginning on page 55 tells the story of the Phoenix Indian Medical Center and its journey to improve medication reconciliation.

When the patient's medications are not relevant to the services provided by your facility, you do not need to document a medication list or reconcile medications.[19] If your facility will prescribe medications, or if the procedure's risk or results might be affected by those medications, then you should ask the patient for a list of current medications.

The Joint Commission's requirement for reconciliation applies to ASCs, ambulatory oncology services, gastrointestinal laboratories, emergency departments, and some imaging procedures. It may not apply, however, to ambulatory settings pursuing routine imaging, laboratory, or physical therapy services. In a walk-in urgent care center, modified medication reconciliation would apply if medication use is part of the facility's services.[19]

It is also important for an ambulatory setting to recognize that it may be called by another health care setting and asked about a patient's list of medications. For instance, if a patient is admitted to an acute care hospital, a staff member may call to ask the primary care physician's staff for an update on the patient's current medications. In general, the clinical staff member who works with the prescribing physician is the one who should be prepared to deliver this information clearly (with read-backs and spell-outs) so that the communication is understood by the other provider. Train staff to request that a complete, updated list be sent to your setting when the patient has been discharged or transferred.[19]

In a clinic or office-based setting, where the patient comes for repeat visits, a complete medication reconciliation should be generated at the initial visit. Thereafter,

the process can simply entail reviewing the list at each visit and updating the list to reflect changes. When other providers of care who are not part of the clinic are involved in the patient's current care, the list should be communicated to them at each update.

Some minimal medication use situations might seem less risky of duplication, omission, or drug interaction.[19] Examples include using topical fluoride in dentistry, local infiltration anesthesia for dental work or suturing lacerations, or enteric barium used in imaging studies. *Minimal use* typically refers to those circumstances in which encounters are in the ambulatory setting, are brief, and do not involve other medication administration, discharge prescription of medications, or any other changes to the patient's current medications. However, there are still scenarios in which the patient's current medications and a list of the patient's drug allergies and past sensitivities should be gathered. Check with the patient, check the documentation, and make an informed decision.

An example is that of propofol (Diprivan). This general anesthetic, which acts as a sedative hypnotic, is a common choice in ambulatory surgical procedures. Sensitivities and allergies to propofol (it contains egg and soy products) can result in adverse effects ranging from local pain on induction to the potentially fatal profolol infusion syndrome. Careful patient history, including a medication reconciliation for this agent, as well as for similarly acting agents such as benzodiazepines and α2-agonists, should always be conducted in office-based and ambulatory surgery centers.[20]

Minimal medication use, calling for a "modified" version of medication reconciliation, involves circumstances in which the following criteria are met[19]:
- There is a brief medical encounter (as mentioned above).
- The medications being administered act locally with negligible systemic effect (for example, minimally absorbed topical agents, low volume local infiltration anesthetics, nonabsorbable enteric contrast agents).
- No other medications are used during the encounter.
- No new medications are prescribed for or given to the patient for use postdischarge.
- There are no changes to the patient's current medications.

■ Any care provider to whom the patient is being referred already has the patient's current medication information.

A two-sided wallet card is available from The Joint Commission for providers to share with patients. These cards provide space for a listing of all the prescription and over-the-counter (OTC) medications that the patient takes to allow him or her to share this information with physicians, nurses, pharmacists, clinical staff, and other caregivers. Staff should encourage patients to carry such a card to prepare them in the event of an untoward medical event. A copy of this card is available on The Joint Commission's Web site .

Modified medication reconciliation can be performed in many ambulatory settings. Assessment tips for the process of medication reconciliation itself are presented in Table 3-7, page 45. When interviewing patients about their medications, use these tips to compile an accurate and complete list.

You don't have to reinvent the wheel to access a standardized form for medication reconciliation. A number of forms are available online and can be modified to meet an individual facility's needs. A useful one-page form has been produced by St. Mary's Medical Center in Green Bay, Wisconsin, which is presented as Figure 3-5, page 48.

Safe Prescription Writing

In a study of four adult primary care practices, one patient developed abdominal discomfort from an excessive dose of hydrocodone/acetaminophen (5/500 tabs; prescribed 12 tabs per day when the recommended maximum is 8 tabs per day).[21] Another patient developed abdominal discomfort from naproxen when he received a prescription intended for another patient. A third patient developed abdominal discomfort from naproxen prescribed at a higher-than-recommended frequency (500 mg, 3 times a day).

Four adult primary care practices in Boston used prescription review, patient survey, and chart review to identify medication errors, potential adverse drug events, preventable adverse drug events, and prescribing errors. These events occurred in 7.6% of outpatient prescriptions, and many of them had the potential to harm patients.[21] In other words, nearly 8 out of every 100 prescriptions written for adults in an ambulatory setting have the potential to become an adverse drug event. Although basic computerized prescribing systems may not be adequate to reduce errors, the authors concluded, future advanced systems with dose and frequency checking may better help to prevent potentially harmful errors. Until the day when all prescribing can be standardized and safeguarded, there are particular risks to prescribing behaviors and systems.

In the study cited above, the most frequent errors on prescriptions were incorrect or missing dose (54%) or frequency (18%). Errors also included prescription rule violations. The most frequent type of error (95%) was a missing administration route (that is, a failure to write "po"). In total, 19% of prescriptions contained either a prescribing error or rule violation. Errors were more likely to occur in the medication classes most commonly prescribed; that is, antibiotics, narcotics, and nonsteroidal anti-inflammatory medications.[21]

✓ Joint Commission requirements call for standardizing a list of abbreviations, acronyms, symbols, and dose designations that are *not* to be used throughout the organization.

Three important elements stand out in the area of safe prescription writing:
1. Avoid dangerous abbreviations.
2. Write clearly and legibly.
3. Include complete information, including stating the purpose for which the medication is being prescribed.

Other risk reduction strategies for safely written prescriptions are presented in Table 3-8, page 50.

Ambiguous medical notations, and some abbreviations, symbols, and dose designations are frequently misinterpreted and lead to mistakes resulting in patient harm. Confusion from misinterpreted handwriting can also delay the start of therapy and waste valuable time spent in clarification.

The Joint Commission "Do Not Use List" is presented in Figure 3-6, page 49.

Safe Use of Sample Medications

Many health care practices supply patients with phar-

Figure 3-5. Outpatient Home Medication Reconciliation Tool

Information Source: ☐ Patient ☐ Clinic Record ☐ Retail Pharmacy_____

☐ Family/Caregiver ☐ SNF/CBRF ☐ Other

Medication	Strength	Dose	Route	Frequency	Used for	Last Dose Date/Time	Discharge Continue	Stop
			☐ Oral ☐ Other	☐ Daily ☐ Twice a day ☐ Three times/day ☐ Other				
			☐ Oral ☐ Other	☐ Daily ☐ Twice a day ☐ Three times/day ☐ Other				
			☐ Oral ☐ Other	☐ Daily ☐ Twice a day ☐ Three times/day ☐ Other				
			☐ Oral ☐ Other	☐ Daily ☐ Twice a day ☐ Three times/day ☐ Other				
			☐ Oral ☐ Other	☐ Daily ☐ Twice a day ☐ Three times/day ☐ Other				
			☐ Oral ☐ Other	☐ Daily ☐ Twice a day ☐ Three times/day ☐ Other				

Allergies **None** **Yes** **(list all)** **Reactions** **Self-Prescribed Medications (Herbals, Supplements, etc.)**

_____ _____ _____

_____ _____ _____

Signature: _____ Date/Time: _____

Signature: _____ Date/Time: _____

Signature: _____ Date/Time: _____

We recommend that you contact your primary health care provider to ensure the medication list is complete and accurate.

Copy to patient and Original to chart

This form is used in high-volume ambulatory areas at two hospitals. To use in a setting that requires a modified medication reconciliation process, the columns "Medication," "Strength," "Dose," and "Used for" would be sufficient.

Source: St. Mary's Medical Center and St. Vincent Hospital, Green Bay, WI. Used with permission.

Figure 3-6. Do Not Use List

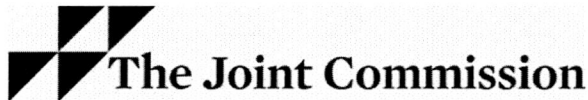

◤◤ The Joint Commission

Official "Do Not Use" List[1]

Do Not Use	Potential Problem	Use Instead
U (unit)	Mistaken for "0" (zero), the number "4" (four) or "cc"	Write "unit"
IU (International Unit)	Mistaken for IV (intravenous) or the number 10 (ten)	Write "International Unit"
Q.D., QD, q.d., qd (daily)	Mistaken for each other	Write "daily"
Q.O.D., QOD, q.o.d, qod (every other day)	Period after the Q mistaken for "I" and the "O" mistaken for "I"	Write "every other day"
Trailing zero (X.0 mg)* Lack of leading zero (.X mg)	Decimal point is missed	Write X mg Write 0.X mg
MS	Can mean morphine sulfate or magnesium sulfate	Write "morphine sulfate" Write "magnesium sulfate"
MSO_4 and $MgSO_4$	Confused for one another	

[1] Applies to all orders and all medication-related documentation that is handwritten (including free-text computer entry) or on pre-printed forms.

*Exception: A "trailing zero" may be used only where required to demonstrate the level of precision of the value being reported, such as for laboratory results, imaging studies that report size of lesions, or catheter/tube sizes. It may not be used in medication orders or other medication-related documentation.

Additional Abbreviations, Acronyms and Symbols
(For <u>possible</u> future inclusion in the Official "Do Not Use" List)

Do Not Use	Potential Problem	Use Instead
> (greater than) < (less than)	Misinterpreted as the number "7" (seven) or the letter "L"	Write "greater than" Write "less than"
	Confused for one another	
Abbreviations for drug names	Misinterpreted due to similar abbreviations for multiple drugs	Write drug names in full
Apothecary units	Unfamiliar to many practitioners	Use metric units
	Confused with metric units	
@	Mistaken for the number "2" (two)	Write "at"
cc	Mistaken for U (units) when poorly written	Write "mL" or "ml" or "milliliters" ("mL" is preferred)
μg	Mistaken for mg (milligrams) resulting in one thousand-fold overdose	Write "mcg" or "micrograms"

These guidelines from The Joint Commission's "Do Not Use" List should be posted and discussed with all staff.

Source: The Joint Commission. http://www.jointcommission.org/PatientSafety/DoNotUseList/ (accessed May 18, 2009).

Table 3-8. Risk Reduction Strategies for Safe Prescription Writing

- Print prescriptions c l e a r l y, LEGIBLY, and indelibly.
- Identify patient's full name, address, and date of birth on the prescription. For pediatric (under 12 years) prescriptions, include child's age and weight.
- Write the international approved drug name in uppercase **BLOCK LETTERS**.
- Do not use chemical descriptions or abbreviations for drug names because they increase the risk of medication errors (for example, $FeSO_4$ or ISMN is not acceptable).
- The bioavailability of some medications may vary between different brands, and these should be prescribed by brand name. Such drugs include, for example, aminophylline modified release, cyclosporine, diltiazem long-acting formulations, lithium, nifedipine, theophylline modified release.
- Use the brand name, where appropriate, in addition to the approved name to avoid confusion.
- In cases of different formulations or strengths of a preparation, when they are available, correctly state the details on the prescription (for example, phenytoin suspension 30 mg/5 mL or 90 mg/5 mL).
- For medication such as insulin and inhalers that are supplied through a device, again, state any details that will ensure that the patient receives the correct product.
- The *dose* must be stated on all prescriptions.
- Avoid unnecessary use of decimal points; for example, 3 mg (not 3.0 mg).
- Quantities of 1 gram or more should be written as 1 g and so on.
- Quantities of less than 1 gram should be written in milligrams, for example, 500 mg (not 0.5 g).
- Quantities of less than 1 milligram should be written in micrograms, for example, 100 micrograms (not 0.1 mg).
- When decimal points are unavoidable, a zero must be put in front of the decimal point when there is no other figure; for example, 0.5 mL (not .5 mL).
- Micrograms, nanograms, and units must be written out fully, not abbreviated.
- g (grams), mg (milligrams), and ml (milliliters), are acceptable abbreviations. Use the upper case L in milliliters (mL).
- Always state the concentration of liquid preparations.
- Specify the route of administration. Be careful when prescribing for different routes because doses may not be equivalent. In such a case, separate prescriptions for each route. (For example, the intravenous dose of morphine is one quarter to one half of the intramuscular dose.)
- Specify directions. State the dose frequency on all prescriptions. For "as required" medications, specify a minimum dose interval and where appropriate, a maximum dose. (For example, write "paracetamol/acetaminophen 500 mg tablets, one to two tablets every four to six hours when required, maximum 8 tablets in 24 hours, for the relief of pain or fever.")
- State the indication for any "as required" medication.
- Where a limited course of treatment is required, state as such on the prescription.
- Include the prescriber's signature and the date and a contact number.

Source: National Health Service, United Kingdom, Wales. http://www.wales.nhs.uk/sites3/Documents/501/AllWRxGuide.doc (accessed May 18, 2009).

TIPS

To further help in reducing medication errors, apply safe prescription-writing and verbal telephone order practices with the patient.

- Spell aloud the name of the drug.
- Clearly inform your patient in the medical encounter regarding the purpose of the drug/agent.
- Advise the patient to read the prescription's accompanying patient leaflet. Many tragic situations could be prevented if the patient would just read the leaflet.

maceutical samples. This is a beneficial practice because it allows the patient to know whether the drug is effective and if it will cause any adverse effects. Security and access are important aspects of supplying sample medications to patients. Just as with larger quantities of medications, samples are subject to safe storage and security principles, including proper light and temperature, segregation of confusing and error-prone dosages and dosage forms, and dispensing documentation. All dispensing and administration standards and elements of performance also apply to sample medications.

Particular risks of dispensing sample medications in an ambulatory setting include the following:

- A pharmacist is not available to fully educate the patient.
- Staff may improperly dispense samples (by dose, drug name, or drug use) without physician oversight.
- Prescription labels for samples may be presigned by physicians.
- Samples may be outdated.
- Drug cabinets are seldom secure.
- Staff or others passing through the area hallways may initiate self-therapy without the supervision of a clinician.

To prevent errors and risks related to sample drugs in your facility, first begin with an assessment, which includes answering the following questions[22]:

- Are your sample drugs organized in a secure cabinet or room?
- Is access limited to qualified staff?
- Is there a lock system in place to restrict access?
- Are sample drugs logged in by pharmaceutical firm representatives?
- Are clinicians provided with drug information to provide to patients regarding safe use of the drug?
- Is a log out system in place such that inventory can be checked?
- Can the log out system be made available in duplicate or triplicate? For example, the first copy can be entered in a sample computer database, the second copy in the patient medical record, and the third sent home with the patient.[23] (Depending on state laws, this last copy might include areas for detailed instructions on the proper way to take medications and any potential side effects.)
- How are drug recalls handled?
- Does someone track all medications in the sample storage site to eliminate outdated drugs?
- Does the cabinet contain drugs that are not utilized and should be eliminated?
- Are LASA issues accommodated?

The National Coordinating Council on Medication Error Reporting and Prevention has an entire set of recommendations related to the safe use of sample medications (*see* http://www.nccmerp.org/council/council2008-01.html).

At Gundersen Lutheran Health System in LaCrosse, Wisconsin, each department has a sign-in/sign-out log for drug reps to use during each visit. They enter the name, medication delivered, lot numbers, quantity, and expiration date. Clinic staff who remove samples sign them out in the same log.[22] Regular reassessment of this process is performed on a monthly basis.

A case study presenting an example of how data tracking and outcomes monitoring of patients' narcotics use helped maintain community safety appears online at http://www.jcrinc.com/PSAC09/extras/.

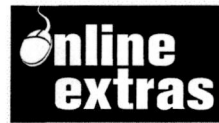

online extras

References

1. Zed P.J., et al.: Incidence, severity and preventability of medication-related visits to the emergency department: A prospective study. *CMAJ* 178:1563–1569, Jun. 3, 2008.
2. National Coordinating Council for Medication Error Reporting and Prevention: *What Is a Medication Error?* 2009. http://www.nccmerp.org/aboutMedErrors.html (accessed Feb. 25, 2009).
3. The Joint Commission: *Safety in the Operating Room.* Oakbrook Terrace, IL: Joint Commission Resources, 2006.
4. Dillman J.R., et al.: Incidence and severity of acute allergic-like reactions to i.v. nonionic iodinated contrast material in children. *Am J Roentgenol* 188:1643–1647, Jun. 1, 2007.
5. ECRI Institute and Institute for Safe Medication Practices: Contrast-induced nephropathy: Can this iatrogenic complication of iodinated contrast be prevented? *PA-PSRS Patient Safety Advisory.* 4(suppl. 1):1–24, Mar. 30, 2007.
6. Purdue University PharmaTAP: *Anticoagulation Toolkit: Reducing Adverse Drug Events and Potential Adverse Drug Events with Unfractionated Heparin, Low Molecular Weight Heparins and Warfarin.* 2008, http://www.purdue.edu/dp/rche/about/centers/pharamtap.pdf/toolkit.pdf (accessed Feb. 27, 2009).
7. Heckinger E., et al.: Disease management: A mid-decade evolution toward patient safety. *Home Health Care Management & Practice* 18:178–185, Apr. 2006.
8. Sheridan-Leos N., Schulmeister L.: Failure mode and effect analysis: A technique to prevent chemotherapy errors. *Clin J Oncol Nurs* 10:393–398, Jul. 2006.
9. Southern Nevada Health District: *Hepatitis C Investigation.* http://www.southernnevadahealthdistrict.org/hepc-investigation/index.php (accessed Sep. 26, 2009).
10. Ambulatory Surgery Centers. Safe injections stressed after Nevada outbreak. *OR Manager* 24:25–27, May 2008.
11. Centers for Disease Control and Prevention: Transmission of hepatitis B and C viruses in outpatient settings New York, Oklahoma, and Nebraska, 2000–2002. *Morb Mortal Wkly Rep* 52:901–906, Sep. 26, 2003.
12. CDC Foundation, HONOReform Foundation, Sep. 2008.
13. Blanchard J.: Environmental controls; multiuse syringes and needles; patient identification; *Staphylococcus aureus*—Clinical Issues—question and answer. *AORN J* Jun. 2003. http://findarticles.com/p/articles/mi_m0FSL/is_6_77/ai_103379538 (accessed Feb. 26, 2009).

14. Giarrizzo-Wilson S.: Medication packing and labeling. *AORN Journal* Jul. 2007. http://findarticles.com/p/articles/mi_m0FSL/is_1_86/ai_n19448222/ (accessed May 15, 2009).

15. Davis T.C., et al.: Improving patient understanding of prescription drug label instructions. *J Gen Intern Med* 24:57–62, Jan. 2009.

16. Schulmeister L.: Look-alike, sound-alike oncology medications. *Clin J Oncol Nurs* 10:35–41, Feb. 2006.

17. Manno M.S., Hayes D.D.: How medication reconciliation saves lives. *Nursing* 36, Mar. 2006. http://www.nursing2006.com/ (accesses Feb. 16, 2009).

18. Henderson J.: What your ASC needs to know about medication reconciliation. *FOCUS* 44–49, Jan.–Feb. 2008.

19. The Joint Commission: *Medication Reconciliation Handbook.* Oakbrook Terrace, IL: Joint Commission Resources, 2006.

20. Huber D.A.: Use of propofol in gastroenterology practice. *Gastroenterology Nurs* 27:242–243, Sep.–Oct. 2004.

21. Gandhi T.K., et al.: Outpatient prescribing errors and the impact of computerized prescribing. *J Gen Intern Med* 20:837–841, Sep. 2005.

22. Schauberger C., et al.: *Ambulatory Patient Safety Toolkit. Safety Collaborative for the OutPatient Environment (SCOPE), Gundersen Lutheran Health System.* Oct. 2003. http://www.gundluth.org/ (accessed Feb. 9, 2009).

23. Weber R.J.: *The Handbook on Storing and Securing Medications.* Oakbrook Terrace, IL: Joint Commission Resources, 2006.

Case Study: Labeling Medications

CASE STUDY AT A GLANCE

Organization: American Access Care, LLC, Glen Rock, Pennsylvania

Setting: Two state-licensed ambulatory surgery centers (New Jersey and Rhode Island); one state-licensed health care clinic and office surgery center (Florida); twenty (20) outpatient interventional radiology centers

Patient Safety Topic: Safe medication labeling

Accomplishment: No occurrences of medication administration errors or incidents.

The Organization

American Access Care, LLC, operates 23 outpatient interventional radiology centers across 12 states, primarily dedicated to the care of dialysis patients' vascular access needs. Their practitioners include board-certified interventional radiologists, board-certified interventional nephrologists, board-certified vascular surgeons, nurse practitioners, and radiology practitioner assistants.

American Access Care has well-developed and effective safety programs that include education and training, monitoring, data collection, corrective action plans, and reinforcement and reassessment of policies and protocols. Leadership consistently communicates the organization's commitment to safety to staff via newsletters, training, e-mails, and periodic meetings.

The organization's safety program involves a team of multidisciplinary leaders with extensive knowledge of the applicable regulations, best practices, and guidelines, as well as experience in the health care field. Representation from senior-level management provides the staff with visible leadership commitment, which empowers the staff to actively participate in the organization's culture of safety.

Project Beginnings
Project Name and Goals

The informal project name was "Labeling of medications, solutions and containers, on and off the sterile field." The specific goals of this initiative were to do the following:

1. Improve patient safety by decreasing preventable adverse drug events and medication errors.
2. Standardize medication labeling throughout the organization.

As the team prepared for initial accreditation, they determined that the process for labeling medications, solutions, and containers was inconsistent across the organization.

Team Members and Roles

The team consisted of the following individuals: Lisa Faller, director of Compliance and Safety (team leader) and Lisa Petrusky, manager of Quality Assurance. Both worked together to develop a uniform process, policies, forms, and education. They also involved the nurses and physicians who work in the centers with the medication-related processes and procedures. After the two-woman team received feedback from this larger group, they shared the processes with each other to determine best practices.

Project Activity
Project Steps

The steps of the safety initiative were as follows:

- Conduct initial surveys to observe practices in each center. The team used a mock survey tool to identify areas that needed to be improved and/or changed.
- Conduct meetings with leadership and the Safety Committee to review and approve safety initiatives (create policies and protocols, training, tools). The team used the results of the mock survey to devise corrective action plans.
- Conduct initial testing in the centers to ensure proper flow and determine additional areas for improvement. Their "draft" protocols and policies were implemented in the centers.
- Gather feedback from clinical staff. The staff in the centers let the team know if the new processes were effective. They provided feedback on how the process could be improved where needed.

(continued on page 54)

Case Study: Labeling Medications (continued)

- Conduct a second meeting with leadership and the organization's Safety Committee to finalize safety initiatives. After gathering feedback from the staff and leadership, they finalized the best practices for the organization.
- Implement policies, protocols, training, and tools.
- Conduct periodic surveys to ensure compliance with the organization's policy. Consistent monitoring and training is required to ensure that all staff in the organization have knowledge of the company's policies and Joint Commission standards.

The team involved both the organization's leadership and clinical staff in the decision and implementation process. Leadership gave the guidelines, and the clinical staff provided hands-on feedback as to the practicality of implementing the initiative. Because of the lack of available specific ambulatory-based information, and because the organization involved all levels of staff in the decision and implementation process, implementation of initiatives has been very successful.

The Tools Used

The project team developed policies, audit tools, and training materials. Because consistent training and audits have been provided, compliance with improvement initiatives remains high.

Old Process/Plan vs. New

There were no previously outlined process policies, audits, or trainings. The company's policy for labeling medications is reviewed with staff during orientation. Because the company acknowledges that policy interpretations can lead to deviations in practice, it performs periodic checks to ensure safe medication administration practices in its centers. Audit results are communicated to the staff in the center and improvements or additional training is conducted if there is an area of concern. The concentrations of medications are limited in its centers, and it has standardized its labeling process.

Staff Training and Education

Because there are 23 centers across the United States, e-mail, conference calls, Web conferences, and periodic audits by a dedicated multispecialty team were necessary to provide the education and follow-up. The team began by providing information and educating the staff in the centers. They then chose a team of "mock surveyors" to audit each center to follow up and provide reeducation if necessary. Next, they compiled the data and reeducated or adjusted the process from the data collected. The process would then start over, if necessary, or they would continue auditing for continuous compliance.

The Outcome

Measurable Outcome/Lessons Learned

Although there were no measurable outcomes, implementing new policies, procedures, and education now provides consistent applications companywide. Initial training was easier than expected. The team chose a fantastic group that came from various educational backgrounds, including registered nurses and radiology technologists with various educational degrees, to assist with implementing the process.

Overall, the organization learned to always test a new process in a select set of centers before implementing companywide. Training and standardization were the project's biggest obstacles. The team had to ensure that they standardized all training so multiple trainers could be used to implement the process.

The trainers included the centers' regional directors, center managers, the quality assurance manager, and the director of compliance and safety. The professional and educational backgrounds of these individuals included registered nurses, radiology technologists, and health services administration personnel. The training team included staff who have expert knowledge and experience in the ambulatory care environment.

The most critical issue the team found related to their success was to involve multidisciplinary leaders and clinical staff in the decision process.

Case Study: Medication Reconciliation

CASE STUDY AT A GLANCE

Organization: Phoenix Indian Medical Center, HIV Center of Excellence

Setting: Ambulatory Medical Clinic

Patient safety topic: Medication safety through medication reconciliation and intensive medication management for HIV patients.

Accomplishment: Drug interactions have decreased 75% over four years and medication refills have decreased to 0% for the past eight months due to intensive medication reconciliation, bar code technology, and medication management through new clinic processes. The clinic has also achieved the goal of 0.5 clinical interventions per patient per clinic.

The Organization

The Phoenix Indian Medical Center HIV Center of Excellence, Phoenix, Arizona, is a clinically based center for HIV care, treatment, research, and intervention. The center is an Indian Health Service (IHS) program at the Phoenix Indian Medical Center serving the tribal and IHS facilities in the area. The ambulatory medical clinic provides medical care and case management for American Indians and Alaskan Natives who are HIV positive. The HIV Center of Excellence employs one family practitioner (M.D.) specializing in HIV management, two registered nurses/HIV case managers, and one clinical HIV pharmacist (Pharm.D.). One pharmacist position is back-filled from general pharmacy staff for annual leave or other absence, and four other pharmacists are trained to cover. In the organization's safety culture, leadership comes from the top down, yet staff still feel empowered in this model.

Project Beginnings

Prior to 2004, the HIV Center of Excellence clinic was solely the responsibility of the physician. After an incident of a drug interaction went undetected by the physician and central pharmacy staff, the resident pharmacist was invited to the clinic to improve pharmaceutical care. The resident pharmacist is a one-year training position, and a longitudinal HIV rotation was developed to meet the needs of the clinic.

The Medication Safety Project included two overall goals:
1. Prevent dispensing of medications with known drug interactions.
2. Prevent dispensing the wrong medications

Needs Identification and Baseline Measures

Anecdotal information on a "few" drug interactions in HIV patients and a "few" errors in medication "mis-fills" led to a decision to investigate these problems. Specifics included the following:

Drug interactions: A drug interaction between an antiretroviral and a stomach medication was missed. This interaction had the potential of causing harm to the patient by providing a less-than-therapeutic dose of the antiretroviral medication. The interaction was discovered at a follow-up appointment after the patient had been dispensed both medications. Pharmacy was asked to get involved to prevent future problems.

Wrong drug: Antiretroviral drugs have similar names and come in different combinations. Dispensing the wrong medication had occurred and could have led to toxicities or treatment failure.

Team Members and Roles

A Positive Care Team was formed involving the physician (team leader), two registered nurse (R.N.) medical case managers, and the pharmacist, with the goal of improving care and safety.

Project Activity
Project Steps
The steps in the project were as follows:
1. Identify factors that contributed to the errors.
2. Eliminate or at least minimize contributing factors.

Drug interactions: The problem identified was that the HIV medications were new and not yet listed in the IHS drug files. Because these drug files were updated centrally, they were not always accurate.

(continued on page 56)

Case Study: Medication Reconciliation (continued)

Action taken: All new medications are now screened with TWO outside drug interaction screening programs because discrepancies were also found between programs.

Wrong drug: Some medications are combinations and were filled with a different combination (for example, Combivir [zidovudine/lamivudine] was filled with Trizivir [zidovudine/lamivudine/abacavir]).

Action taken: Generic names such as zidovudine/lamivudine/abacavir were changed to their brand names—in this case, Trizivir—on the pharmacy label. All antiretrovirals were filled by the clinical HIV pharmacist when possible. Most recently the newly deployed RxCentral in primary care and main pharmacies prevents filling the wrong medication via bar code recognition software.

The Tools Used

The team used tools available from three interactive drug interaction screening engines:

1. AIDSMEDS (http://www.aidsmeds.com/ cmm) Denver Principles Project (*see* Figure 3-7, below)
2. Micromedex (http://www.micromedex.com) Thomson Reuters Healthcare (*see* Figure 3-8, page 57)
3. UpToDate (http://www.uptodate.com) Lexi-Comp, Inc., accessible through the decision support software UpToDate (available by subscription), (*see* Figures 3-9, page 57, and 3-10, page 58).

Online extras
To view additional tools used for this case study, visit the Online Extras at http://www.jcrinc.com/PSAC09/extras/.

Figure 3-7. Sample Online Drug Interaction Screen

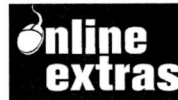

At the AIDSMEDS Web site, medications are registered for each patient by means of online software. This screen allows providers to enter all medications that the patient is taking.

Case Study: Medication Reconciliation (continued)

Figure 3-8. Sample Screen to Analyze Drug Interactions

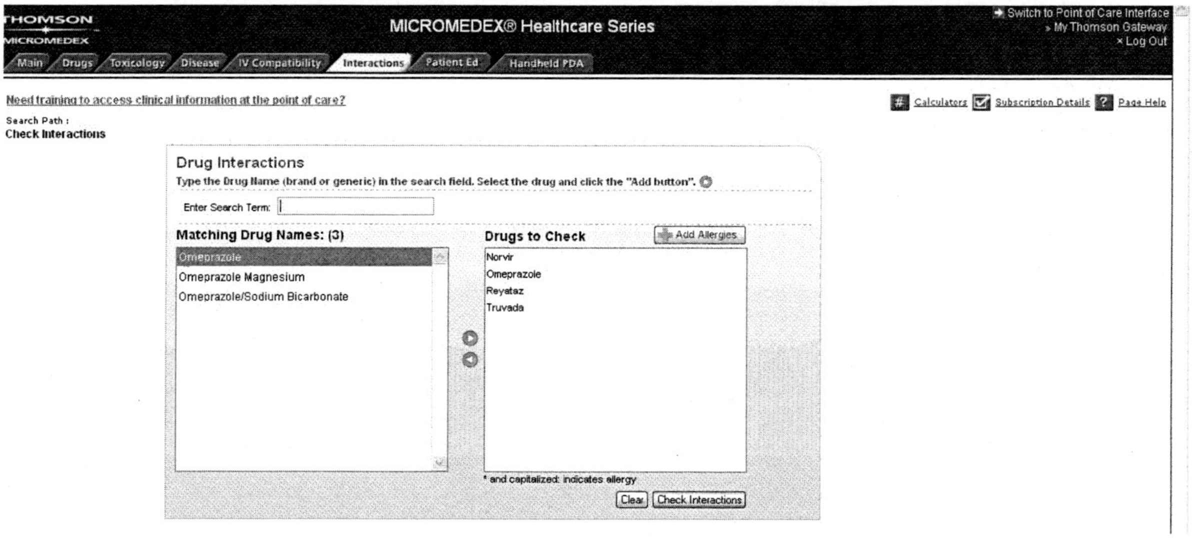

Screens allow interactive searching for drug-drug interactions.

Figure 3-9. Sample Policy Screen

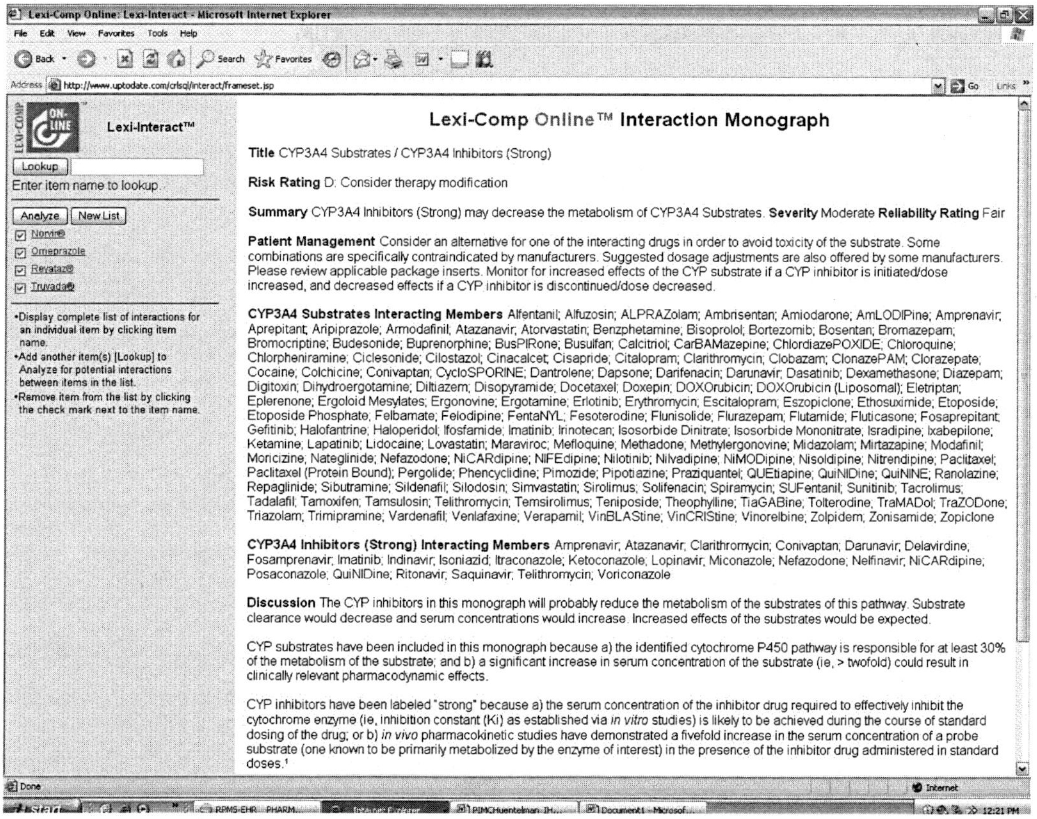

One sign-on screen requests acceptance of policy, which helps maintain patient safety.

(continued on page 58)

Case Study: Medication Reconciliation (continued)

Figure 3-10. Sample Interaction Analysis Introduction Screen

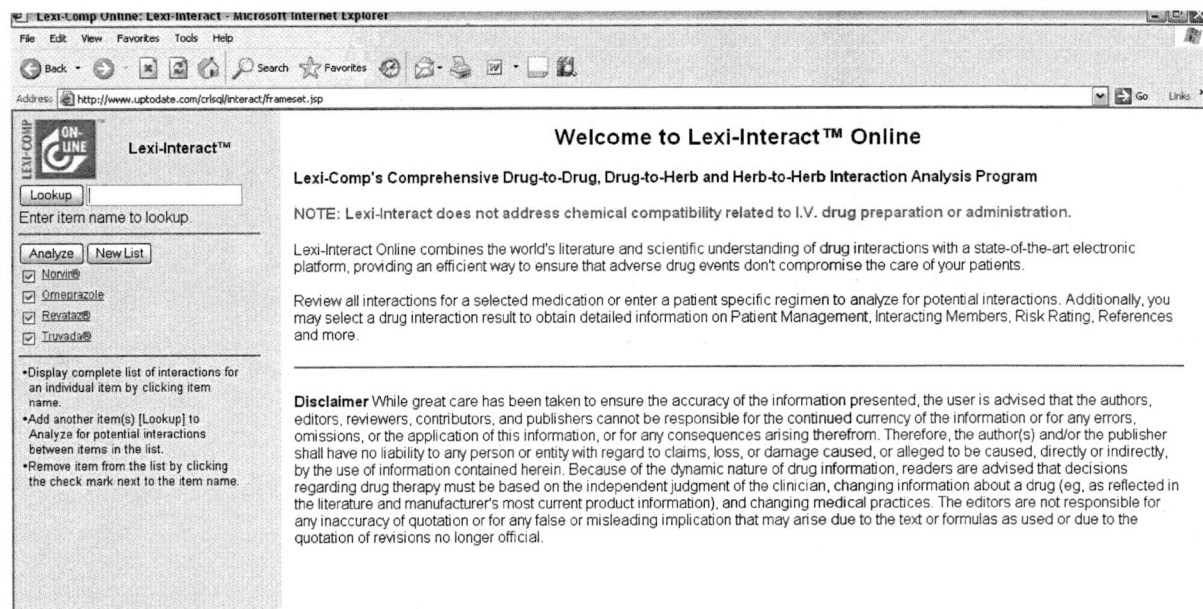

This screen allows the provider to conduct an interactive analysis of interactions with both prescription and nonprescription drugs.

Old Process/Plan vs. New

The new process affects issues of drug interactions and wrong drugs.

Drug interactions: With the old process, staff relied on drug files within the IHS electronic pharmacy system for information on drug interactions. With the new process, staff rely on more current drug files in other resources (listed in "The Tools Used" section) and/or manually update the local pharmacy system with important drug interactions information. The pharmacy package used by IHS has a drug interactions management tool. Drug interactions can be added between agents, and interactions can be flagged at different alert levels. The highest level requires an electronic signature from a pharmacist to continue entering the current medications. If a particular drug interaction seems to be missed, the file can be changed to require an electronic signature, hopefully prompting closer scrutiny and preventing the drug interaction. This has been most commonly used when medications are not contraindicated but require specific spacing or special instructions to prevent a drug interaction.

Wrong drug: In the old process, the prescription was filled by any staff member, including technicians, pharmacists, or pharmacists specially trained in HIV care. In the interim, prescriptions were filled only by an HIV-trained pharmacist during clinic; however, refills were still filled by any staff member. The new process uses the RxCentral® VeriScript® bar code system for identification of relevant information during clinic and for refills in the primary care and main pharmacies. VeriScript® is a dispensing error prevention system that allows pharmacy personnel to confirm that the product selected from the shelf matches the product printed on the prescription label. This process reduces misfills and misbranding, ensuring increased safety for the patient.

Staff Training and Education

The pharmacy resident trained the clinical HIV pharmacists one-on-one regarding the new process. The HIV team discussed errors and prevention methods with all pharmacy staff via meetings and e-mail.

Case Study: Medication Reconciliation (continued)

The Outcome

Measurable Outcomes

Misfilling medications decreased 50% in the first two years with the intervention and filling of prescriptions only by the clinical HIV pharmacist. Misfilling medications decreased to 0% over the past six to eight months with the filling of prescriptions by the clinical HIV pharmacist and filling of medications by the primary care and main pharmacy.

Drug interactions have decreased by 75% due to medication being filled under the new HIV clinic medication management process using outside programs (Micromedex, and so on) to screen for drug interactions.

It should be noted that although misfilling medications and drug interactions have significantly decreased for patients who are managed through the HIV clinic, occasional misfills and drug interactions are observed for patients who obtain their medications from outside clinics and pharmacies and through emergency rooms. Further interventions and actions need to be taken to eliminate or decrease incidents that occur in those areas.

Another outcome was to provide 0.5 clinical interventions per patient per clinic. Interventions include the number and nature of drug interactions, and proper dosing based on information, including lab values. Interventions were logged on a spreadsheet requiring documentation of the type of recommendation, whether it was accepted, and any additional information. Documenting an intervention should take 20 seconds or less. A new electronic intervention system is currently being deployed, and documentation should take about the same amount of time as the paper intervention. The main pharmacy documents about 100 interventions per month with services seven days per week, and inpatient documents more than 200 per month with 24-hour service. The HIV clinic documents 30 interventions per month with 1.5 days of clinic per week, seeing approximately 18 patients per week.

Lessons Learned

The team learned it is important to troubleshoot and test electronic systems before implementing a new system. Drug interaction screenings were tested on different systems, including the newest agents. Known interactions were screened based on information from the package inserts. Results varied slightly depending on the search engine. The team determined it would be best to consult two sources prior to making a clinical decision. This is specific to the HIV medications because the approval process is accelerated, and even the search engines may not be as up to date as another system.

For this team, the full-time equivalent (FTE) to provide the needed pharmaceutical care was the most critical issue that had to be addressed. The HIV clinical pharmacist provided improved safety as an HIV medication expert, preventing drug interactions, dosing errors, and other problems. Staff pharmacists would rely on the expertise of the prescribing physician, and the HIV clinical pharmacist provides the needed double check. The position was funded by the support of administration. In return for a new clinical position, the HIV pharmacist would be charged with decreasing costs of antiretrovirals to Phoenix Indian Medical Center by using patient alternative resources. Phoenix Indian Medical Center is the payer of last resort and hoped to pay only for antiretrovirals for patients without other resources. Since starting in the HIV clinic, the clinical pharmacist has saved the facility 1.3 million dollars over three years. This far exceeds the salary of the new position and has been determined to be a valuable investment for the facility.

The biggest obstacles for achieving success involved updating the current pharmacy drug files. The drug interaction files were not up to date centrally, and updating the files manually at the local level was time consuming and could result in errors. This is why outside drug interaction screening with a combination of selected drug interaction manual entry at the local level was used. RxCentral®, VeriScript®, and the

(continued on page 60)

Case Study: Medication Reconciliation (continued)

other platforms deployed to increase patient safety and pharmacy efficiency were challenging due to the cost of implementation. For instance, the equipment is under lease at $200,000 per year.

Patient acceptance of the new team format went very smoothly. The prior physician in the clinic was very accessible to the individual patient but did not have enough time consistently for all the management required. The case managers and pharmacist are the first point of contact and try to handle problems and refer as needed to the physician. There was concern that patients may have preferred to speak with the physician directly, but patients are just happy to receive the information that they need and do not necessarily care who the contact person is.

Chapter 4

SURGICAL SAFETY

This chapter examines a number of safety issues that must be addressed by ambulatory care organizations that provide surgical services. Included are discussions on anesthesia safety—with a section on preventing and managing malignant hypothermia (MH)—preventing surgical fires, patient burns, and surgical site infections (SSI)s; and preventing wrong-site, wrong-procedure and wrong-person surgery.

Anesthesia Safety

The health care demands of patients and surgeons and an evolving economic environment have led to a surge in both ambulatory surgery centers (ASCs) and office-based surgery (OBS) and, consequently, office-based anesthesia. High-quality office-based anesthesia must be founded in patient safety.

Anesthesia is used in procedures performed in outpatient clinics, ASCs, and OBS settings. Ambulatory anesthesia is tailored to meet the needs of the procedure so that patients may return home shortly after the operation. Short-acting anesthetic drugs and specialized anesthetic techniques can be specifically focused on the needs of the ambulatory patient.

Proactive patient-safety processes in ambulatory anesthesia include attention to preinduction assessments, airway maintenance, intraprocedural monitoring and staffing requirements, intraprocedural sedation level and pain assessment, malignant hypethermia, and postanesthesia monitoring. Information on these areas follows.

Preinduction Assessments

Preinduction assessments before ambulatory surgery should particularly focus on undiagnosed sleep apnea and patient allergies.

Undiagnosed sleep apnea. Obstructive sleep apnea (OSA) is a sleep disorder characterized by recurrent episodes of complete and partial airway collapse during sleep, resulting in apnea (complete absence of breathing lasting more than 10 seconds) or hypoapnea (diminished airflow and oxygen desaturation that occurs for 3 to 10 seconds).[1] OSA can result in a number of adverse effects. It is estimated that 2% to 4% of the U.S. adult population suffers from OSA; approximately 4% of women and 9% of men in the United States (ages 40 to 65) have moderate OSA. About 80% to 90% of OSA patients are undiagnosed. Reasons may include clinicians' inability to recognize sleep-related symptoms and lack of time and resources to perform an all-night sleep study or polysomnogram, the gold standard test for diagnosing OSA.

Identifying OSA patients during the perioperative period may help reduce complications; however, in many ambulatory surgical facilities, preoperative screening focuses on diagnoses of heart and lung disease. Little attention may be given to breathing disorders such as OSA. The initial preoperative screening evaluation is important to reduce the risk of surgical complications from OSA. The preoperative evaluation includes a review of the medical history and a physical examination. The anesthesia provider's review of the patient's health record focuses on any previous airway difficulty with anesthetics, identifying comorbidities associated with OSA, such as hypertension, right heart failure, pulmonary hypertension, diabetes, and arrhythmias. Providers should also consider findings from any sleep studies, if available.

An evaluation of the airway, nasopharyngeal features, neck circumference, tonsil size, and tongue volume should all be included as part of a physical examination. In the absence of a sleep study's results, a presumptive diagnosis of OSA may be made based on the patient's medical history, a physical assessment, and clinical symptoms identified during the interviews or by a screening tool. A useful screening tool for OSA is presented in Figure 4-1, page 62.

As identified by the American Society of Anesthesiologists (ASA) Task Force on Perioperative

Figure 4-1. Obstructive Sleep Apnea Preoperative Screening Tool

This questionnaire is a sample tool to screen for obstructive sleep apnea. It is not a substitute for a sleep disorder evaluation by a qualified physician. However, it may help identify at-risk patients during the preoperative period.

Answer YES or NO to each question and place an "X" in the corresponding column.
(To be completed by the patient and his or her bedroom partner.)

Questions	Yes	No
1. Do you snore loudly (e.g., can you be heard through a closed door)?	___	___
2. Does your bedroom partner complain about your snoring?	___	___
3. Does your snoring wake you up at night?	___	___
4. Do you or your bedroom partner notice that you make gasping and choking noises during sleep?	___	___
5. Has your bedroom partner ever noticed that you have stopped breathing during sleep for 10 to 30 seconds?	___	___
6. Do you have a dry mouth, sore throat, or headache in the morning?	___	___
7. Do you often fall asleep during the daytime when you want to stay awake?	___	___
8. Are you often tired during the day?	___	___
9. Have you ever been told that you have obstructive sleep apnea?	___	___

ALERT ANESTHESIA if patient answers YES to any of the above.

This preoperative tool can help you identify patients at risk for OSA.

Source: ECRI Institute and Institute for Safe Medication Practices: Obstructive sleep apnea may block the path to a positive postoperative outcome. *PA-PSRS Patient Safety Advisory* 4:91, Sep. 2007.

Management of Obstructive Sleep Apnea, patients with documented or suspected OSA may be candidates for ambulatory surgery if they have OSA that does not require continuous positive airway pressure, will undergo a minimally invasive procedure, will be administered only a local anesthetic, or will have a limited need for narcotic analgesia.

Allergies. Prior to surgery, the patient should be asked about any medication allergies, including those revealed by previous surgeries. This should be noted in the medical record. As a safeguard, before any medication is administered during the surgical procedure, a designated staff member should once again verify the patient's identity and check the medical record for allergies.

A wise step is to query staff with a proactive risk assessment to determine if the organization has any problems in obtaining, documenting, and quickly retrieving allergy information.[2] Some tips for handling allergies are listed in Table 4-1, page 63.

Airway Maintenance

Respiratory events are the second most common adverse event associated with anesthesia, with an approximate frequency of 1%.[3] Although severe allergic reactions to contrast material are rare in both adults and children, staff must be competent to respond to these events in ambulatory settings. Simulation is a growing tool in medicine and allows standardized exposure of trainees to uncommon events in a setting that is conducive to education without fear of repercussions. Simulation exercises also provide patient-safety practice and education without putting patients at risk.[4,5]

Intraprocedural Monitoring and Staffing Requirements

If your facility provides anesthesia in the course of patient care, policy must dictate provider privileges for administering and monitoring minimal sedation, moderate sedation, and deep sedation (and general anesthesia). Granting of privileges should be made according to strict standards approved by academic specialty societies such as the American Academy of Pediatrics and the American Society of Anesthesiologists.[6]

The ambulatory medical practice or center should implement and maintain a system to do the following[7]:

■ Periodically (at least annually) conduct an assessment of all nursing and support staff for competency that is sufficient and appropriate for the services and procedures they perform.

■ Educate employees about new drugs and products before they are prescribed or used by the practice.

■ Provide continuing education to clinical and support personnel that is both specific and appropriate for the level of services provided in the practice.

A good template for developing a policy and outlining staffing requirements is provided in the instrument available online from Children's Hospital and Health System, Inc., a consortium of inpatient and outpatient facilities in Wisconsin (http://www.chw. org).[6]

Intraprocedural Sedation Level and Pain Assessment

Anesthesia-induced unconsciousness is accompanied by physiologic deterioration and increased patient risk.[6] Minimal sedation, moderate sedation, deep sedation, and general anesthesia are descriptions of arbitrary points along a continuum of unconsciousness in which progressive loss of protective reflexes produces progressive increase in physiologic change and potential risk to the patient.[8]

A standardized preprocedural risk assessment should be conducted with the patient and a full medical history. The ASA classification system is used to identify patients at risk of anesthesia complications. This classi-

---

> ### Table 4-1. Tips for Risk Reduction in Treating Patients with Medication Allergies
>
> ■ Designate a specific place in the medical record for allergy information. Electronic medical records can make this particularly easy.
> ■ During a surgical procedure, continually monitor the patient's response to any administered medication for evidence of an adverse reaction.
> ■ Document sensitivities or allergies to chemicals and reagents such as formalin, saline, radiopaque, dyes, and glutaraldehyde in the same standardized way as medications.

fication is presented in Table 4-2, page 65.

Malignant Hyperthermia

Every surgical organization must have policies in place for dealing with emergencies in patient care. One of the most important aspects of anesthesia asfety is the organization's plan for (and ability to) manage the development of malignant hyperthermia (MH).

As defined by the Malignant Hyperthermia Association of the United States (MHAUS), "Malignant hyperthermia is an inherited disorder of skeletal muscle triggered in susceptibles (human or animal) in most instances by inhalation agents, and/or succinylcholine resulting in hypermetabolism, skeletal muscle damage, hyperthermia and death if untreated."

The effectiveness of diagnostic testing options to evaluate MH susceptibility depends on the pretest probability that the patient is MH susceptible. Diagnostic tests are most useful when making treatment decisions for surgical patients for whom the probability of MH susceptibility is high.[9]

MH trigger agents include potent volatile anesthetics such as halothane, sevoflurane, desflurane, and succinylcholine. Agents that are not triggers for MH include intravenous agents, nondepolarizing agents, ketamine, propofol, and anxiolytics. MHAUS advises that before any diagnostic testing is performed, the patient should be evaluated for susceptibility to MH using available medical data. Because susceptibility to MH is inherited from an autosomal dominant gene, carefully review the medical histories of patients as well as their family members for genetic risk factors.[9,10]

Figure 4-2. Emergency Therapy for Malignant Hyperthermia

Effective May 2008

MH Hotline
1-800-644-9737
Outside the US:
1-315-464-7079

EMERGENCY THERAPY FOR
MALIGNANT HYPERTHERMIA

DIAGNOSIS vs. ASSOCIATED PROBLEMS

Signs of MH:
- Increasing ETCO₂
- Trunk or total body rigidity
- Masseter spasm or trismus
- Tachycardia/tachypnea
- Mixed Respiratory and Metabolic Acidosis
- Increased temperature (may be late sign)
- Myoglobinuria

Sudden/Unexpected Cardiac Arrest in Young Patients:
- Presume hyperkalemia and initiate treatment (see #6)
- Measure CK, myoglobin, ABGs, until normalized
- Consider dantrolene
- Usually secondary to occult myopathy (e.g., muscular dystrophy)
- Resuscitation may be difficult and prolonged

Trismus or Masseter Spasm with Succinylcholine
- Early sign of MH in many patients
- If limb muscle rigidity, begin treatment with dantrolene
- For emergent procedures, continue with non-triggering agents, evaluate and monitor the patient, and consider dantrolene treatment
- Follow CK and urine myoglobin for 36 hours.
- Check CK immediately and at 6 hour intervals until returning to normal. Observe for dark or cola colored urine. If present, liberalize fluid intake and test for myoglobin
- Observe in PACU or ICU for at least 12 hours

ACUTE PHASE TREATMENT

1 GET HELP. GET DANTROLENE – Notify Surgeon
- Discontinue volatile agents and succinylcholine.
- Hyperventilate with 100% oxygen at flows of 10 L/min. or more.
- Halt the procedure as soon as possible; if emergent, continue with non-triggering anesthetic technique.
- Don't waste time changing the circle system and CO₂ absorbant.

2 Dantrolene 2.5 mg/kg rapidly IV through large-bore IV, if possible

To convert kg to lbs for amount of dantrolene, give patients 1 mg/lb (2.5 mg/kg approximates 1 mg/lb).

- Dissolve the 20 mg in each vial with at least 60 ml sterile, preservative-free water for injection. Prewarming (not to exceed 39° C.) the sterile water may expidite solubilization of dantrolene. However, to date, there is no evidence that such warming improves clinical outcome.
- Repeat until signs of MH are reversed.
- Sometimes more than 10 mg/kg (up to 30 mg/kg) is necessary.

- Each 20 mg bottle has 3 gm mannitol for isotonicity. The pH of the solution is 9.

3 Bicarbonate for metabolic acidosis
- 1-2 mEq/kg if blood gas values are not yet available.

4 Cool the patient with core temperature >39°C. Lavage open body cavities, stomach, bladder, or rectum. Apply ice to surface. Infuse cold saline intravenously. Stop cooling if temp. <38°C and falling to prevent drift < 36°C.

5 Dysrhythmias usually respond to treatment of acidosis and hyperkalemia.
- Use standard drug therapy **except calcium channel blockers, which may cause hyperkalemia or cardiac arrest in the presence of dantrolene.**

6 Hyperkalemia – Treat with hyperventilation, bicarbonate, glucose/insulin, calcium.
- Bicarbonate 1-2 mEq/kg IV.
- For **pediatric**, 0.1 units insulin/kg and 1 ml/kg 50% glucose or for **adult**, 10 units regular insulin IV and 50 ml 50% glucose.
- Calcium chloride 10 mg/kg or calcium gluconate 10-50 mg/kg for life-threatening hyperkalemia.
- Check glucose levels hourly.

7 Follow ETCO₂, electrolytes, blood gases, CK, core temperature, urine output and color, coagulation studies. If CK and/or K+ rise more than transiently or urine output falls to less than 0.5 ml/kg/hr, induce diuresis to >1 ml/kg/hr and give bicarbonate to alkalinize urine to prevent myoglobinuria-induced renal failure. (See D below)
- Venous blood gas (e.g., femoral vein) values may document hypermetabolism better than arterial values.
- Central venous or PA monitoring as needed and record minute ventilation.
- Place Foley catheter and monitor urine output.

POST ACUTE PHASE

A Observe the patient in an ICU for at least 24 hours, due to the risk of recrudescence.
B Dantrolene 1 mg/kg q 4-6 hours or 0.25 mg/kg/hr by infusion for at least 24 hours. Further doses may be indicated.
C Follow vitals and labs as above (see #7)
- Frequent ABG as per clinical signs
- CK every 8-12 hours; less often as the values trend downward

D Follow urine myoglobin and institute therapy to prevent myoglobin precipitation in renal tubules and the subsequent development of Acute Renal Failure. CK levels above 10,000 IU/L is a presumptive sign of rhabdomyolysis and myoglobinuria. Follow standard intensive care therapy for acute rhabdomyolysis and myoglobinuria (urine output >2 ml/kg/hr by hydration and diuretics along with alkalinization of urine with Na-bicarbonate infusion with careful attention to both urine and serum pH values).
E Counsel the patient and family regarding MH and further precautions; refer them to MHAUS. Fill out and send in the Adverse Metabolic Reaction to Anesthesia (AMRA) form (www.mhreg.org) and send a letter to the patient and her/his physician. Refer patient to the nearest Biopsy Center for follow-up.

Non-Emergency Information
MHAUS
PO Box 1069 (11 East State Street)
Sherburne, NY 13460-1069
Phone
1-800-986-4287
(607-674-7901)
Fax
607-674-7910
Email
info@mhaus.org
Website
www.mhaus.org

Since 1981
Dedicated to Patient Safety

CAUTION: This protocol may not apply to all patients; alter for specific needs.

Modify this poster as necessary for your individual facility.

Source: Malignant Hyperthermia Association of the United States.

Table 4-2. ASA Classification of Sedation

ASA Class	Definition
I	A normal, healthy patient
II	A patient with mild systemic disease and no functional limitations (such as tobacco use, controlled hypertension, or controlled diabetes)
III	A patient with moderate to severe systemic disease that results in some functional limitations (for example, patients with chronic obstructive pulmonary disease, asthma, congestive heart failure, chronic renal failure, or uncontrolled diabetes)
IV	A patient with severe systemic disease that is a constant threat to life and is functionally incapacitating (such as metastatic cancer or cardiomyopathy)

Source: American Society of Anesthesiologists.

Sidebar 4-1. Diagnostic Tests for Malignant Hyperthermia (MH)

Available Diagnostic Tests for MH:
- Muscle Contracture Test: Caffeine Halothane Contracture Test (CHCT). CHCT is a method of contracture testing performed in North America, while IVCT (In Vitro Contracture Testing) is the method of contracture testing performed in Europe and some other countries. This is the most sensitive and specific diagnostic test for MH susceptibility.
- Genetic Testing (Ryanodine Receptor [RYR1] gene sequencing)

CHCT Test Indications
- Patient with a relative with known genetic susceptibility (as determined by positive muscle contracture test)
- Patient with a family history that suggests MH (as determined by past suspicious MH episode in a family member, but without a known RYR1 causative genetic mutation)
- Patient with past suspected MH event (wait 3–6 months postevent, depending on the degree of rhabdomyolysis). (Rhabdomyolysis is the breakdown of muscle fibers causing the release of muscle fiber contents [myoglobin] into the bloodstream. Some of these contents threaten the kidney and often result in kidney damage.)
- Patient with severe Masseter muscle rigidity (MMR) during anesthesia with a triggering agent
- Patient with moderate to mild MMR with evidence of rhabdomyolysis
- Patient with unexplained rhabdomyolysis during or after surgery (may present as sudden cardiac arrest due to hyperkalemia)
- Patient with exercise-induced rhabdomyolysis after a negative rhabdomyolysis workup
- Signs suggestive of but not definitive for MH
- If military service is desired, patients with suspicion of MH susceptibility are required to undergo CHCT.

Source: Malignant Hyperthermia Association of the United States: MHAUS Guidelines. Testing for Malignant Hyperthermia (MH) Susceptibility: How do I counsel my patients?

Available diagnostic tests and testing indications are presented in Sidebar 4-1 on this page.

Emergency therapy for MH is outlined in the poster presented in Figure 4-2, page 64, which is available for download at the MHAUS Web site, http://www.mhaus.org. A case study describing the development of a MH response begins on page 72.

Post-anesthesia Monitoring

The American Association of Nurse Anesthetists considers the surgical postanesthesia period as an extension of the anesthesia process and that the anesthesia care provider's responsibility to the patient extends through this period. In all practice settings, this responsibility includes a thorough knowledge of the patient's needs, the communication of those needs to qualified providers, and the assurance that the postanesthesia care will be consistent with the patient's needs.

Patient Falls

Although the risk of patient falls is receiving a concerted effort for patient safety initiatives in hospitals, ambulatory settings are not immune to this risk. Falls are an issue for patients undergoing ambulatory procedures or surgery because the vast majority of patients receive sedatives, anesthetics, or pain medications as part of their care. Using these medications increases the possibility of a fall. *See* "Patient Assessments" in Chapter 7, "Staff Education and Training," for a discussion of this topic.

Emergency Power Sources

As part of a comprehensive emergency management plan (*see* Chapter 6, "Environment and Equipment"), every ambulatory organization needs a contingency plan for emergency power sources when normal power sources are unavailable.[11] Such considerations are paramount to conserve basic life support and sustain the application of anesthesia.

Table 4-3. Steps in Planning a Fire Drill

Three months in advance
- Develop a detailed scenario so that everyone understands the plan.
- Develop a time line of drill events to ensure that everything is accomplished in a timely fashion.
- Establish the exact date and time for the fire drill.

Two months in advance
- Review organization fire drill evaluation forms and make minor adjustments to them as needed.
- Identify two individuals to act as fire coordinators.
- Identify individuals (for example, service coordinators, computer system specialist, risk managers, chief anesthesia care provider, endoscopy and sterile processing managers) to observe three to four operating rooms (ORs) during the drill.
- Designate locations for each observer.
- Plan a debriefing meeting to evaluate the drill.

One month in advance
- Designate one person to be stationed at the telephone to schedule any emergency procedures.
- Designate and notify one surgical team to be available if an emergency procedure is scheduled.
- Review fire safety information with OR staff members at a staff member conference.

Two weeks in advance
- Notify surgical executive team members of the drill plan.
- Make signs to identify individuals who are observers so that staff members will not ask for their assistance.
- Post signs to remind everyone of the upcoming drill.

One week in advance
- Notify organization executive team members and the local fire department of the drill plan.
- Notify organization directors and managers of the drill to avoid undue concern when the fire alarms sound.
- Explain to non–OR staff members where they should be and what their role is in the drill.
- Distribute observer signs to the observers.
- Review the drill plan with staff members.
- Review evaluation worksheets with staff members.

One day in advance
- Obtain CPR mannequins to simulate patients for procedures that require complex patient positioning.

The day of the drill
- Briefly review drill information with staff members and answer any questions.
- Provide each emergency team member with a portable telephone to facilitate communication.
- Place stretchers by each OR to simulate a busy hallway.
- Enact the fire drill at 6:30 A.M. or at the start of the morning, before patients arrive.

After the drill
- Hold a debriefing session with managers to discuss the fire drill.
- Report information gleaned from the debriefing session to OR staff members.
- Give items (that is, evaluation worksheets) used in the fire drill to risk management personnel.

Source: Adapted from Salmon L.: Fire in the OR—Prevention and preparedness. *AORN J* 80:42–48, 51–54, Jul. 2004.

Questions to ask regarding emergency needs are whether a two-way communication source, which is not dependent on electrical current, is available and whether the location has sufficient electrical outlets to power all anesthesia machines and monitoring equipment. Organizations should also arrange for a secondary power source, as appropriate for equipment in use, in case of power failure. Clearly label outlets and connections to an emergency power supply. These steps should be noted as part of a preoperative checklist, or a designated provider, such as the certified nurse anesthetist if there is one at the site, should be cited as accountable for backup plans.

All ASCs and OBS settings should explore with reputable vendors a system that will best meet the organization's needs. Considerations should include how long such a system should be capable of providing power.[11] Klein and Ginsberg supply a list of useful resources for ASCs on applicable standards as well as a list of local, federal, and nongovernmental organizations with information on this topic.[11]

TOOL: Emergency Management and Fire Drills

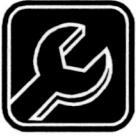

Preparedness for emergencies, including fires, requires proactive planning. Below are tools that can be used for evacuation from fires or other threats.

Rex Healthcare System in Raleigh, North Carolina, used specific forms during and after a fire drill for their 12-room same-day surgery unit (as well as their 300-bed community hospital).[12] Prior to the drill, the surgical services staff identified teams, designated leaders, and met to coordinate activities, and developed a time frame for the time allowed for each task. Table 4-3, page 66, includes the steps they used to plan and execute a fire drill. After each drill or event, management reviews the evaluations and plans and conducts in-service programs accordingly. At Rex, 90% is the minimum passing evaluation score.[12]

Surgical Fires

✔ Joint Commission requirements call for organizations to educate staff, including licensed independent practitioners who are involved with surgical procedures, and anesthesia providers, on how to control heat sources and how to manage fuels while maintaining enough time for patient preparation, and to establish guidelines to minimize oxygen concentration under surgical drapes.

Fires taking place during a surgical procedure are a serious danger for patients and operating room (OR) staff. According to estimates from ECRI and the U.S. Food and Drug Administration, as published in a guideline statement of the Association of PeriOperative Registered Nurses (AORN), approximately 100 surgical fires (some 2 each week) occur annually.[13] These result in about 20 serious patient injuries and 1 to 2 deaths per year.

Of the OR fires that have been reported, 68% of ignition sources originate from electrosurgical units, 13% involve lasers, and other fires originate from electrocautery equipment, fiberoptic light, defibrillators, and high-speed burs, which can produce sparks.[13]

Moreover, in 78% of fires, the presence of oxygen-enriched atmospheres was involved.

A fire prevention program involves four steps: established objectives, a well-prepared management team, best practices outlines, and education and training.[13] Certain equipment and supplies must be available in every surgical suite and procedure room for emergency response. Supplies that should be immediately available in case of fire include the following[14]:

- CO_2 fire extinguisher
- Replacement tracheal tubes, guides, facemasks
- Rigid laryngoscope blades (may include a rigid fiberoptic laryngoscope)
- Replacement airway breathing circuits and lines
- Replacement drapes, sponges

The PASS procedures[15] provides a mnemonic on how to properly operate a fire extinguisher:
1. **P**ull the pin, release a lock latch, or press a puncture lever.
2. **A**im the extinguisher nozzle, horn, or nose at the base of the fire.
3. **S**queeze or press the handle.
4. **S**weep from side-to-side in most cases. But extinguishing techniques vary. Read the directions.

Patient Burns

Patient burns may or may not result from OR fires. In addition to the other tips and techniques for preventing and handling OR fires listed elsewhere in this chapter, suggested responses to patient burns involving a surgical wound or the patient's airway are listed in Table 4-4, page 68. Take these actions immediately in the event of a surgical wound or patient airway fire.

Surgical Site Infections

✔ Joint Commission requirements call for instituting best practices to prevent surgical site infections.

To prevent surgical site infections (SSIs) in ambulatory health care (AHC), perioperative care includes appropriate use of antibiotics, appropriate hair removal, and perioperative normothermia. Postoperative SSIs are a major source of illness in outpatients, accounting for between about 25% and 40% of health care–acquired infections each year.[16,17]

An SSI is defined as one of three classifications:
1. Superficial incisional infection
2. Deep incisional infection
3. Infection of the organ or space

The Centers for Disease Control and Prevention (CDC) use the criteria presented in Table 4-5, page 69, to define SSIs in these three standardized categories.

In 1999 the CDC's Health Care Infection Control Practices Advisory Committee published revised guidelines for the prevention of SSIs.[18] Sidebar 4-2, page·70, presents a summary of preventive practices for reducing these infections. These practices can help ASCs and OBS practices meet Joint Commission National Patient Safety Goal 7.

Wrong-Person, Wrong-Site, Wrong-Side, Wrong-Procedure, or Wrong-Implant Surgery

Wrong-site surgery would seem to be a rare concern in the ambulatory setting, but it does occur, particularly if general anesthetics or conscious sedation is provided. The Joint Commission's Universal Protocol for Preventing Wrong Site, Wrong Procedure and Wrong Person Surgery™ addresses use of a preoperative checklist, marking the surgical site on the patient, and providing for effective time-outs. Strategies to maintain safety first, without interrupting or delaying patient flow, are also an important part of the protocol.

As of April 10, 2009, the Universal Protocol 2009 has been endorsed by more than 20 national membership associations and organizations. The Universal Protocol addresses the continuing occurrence of wrong-site, wrong-procedure and wrong-person surgery in Joint Commission–accredited hospitals, ambulatory care organizations, and OBS facilities. The Universal Protocol drew on, and expanded and integrated, a series of requirements under The Joint Commission's National Patient Safety Goals. An updated Universal Protocol became effective January 1, 2009. The elements of the Universal Protocol, which is undergoing examination and may be revised in the next year or two, are listed in Sidebar 4-3, page 71.

Using a preoperative checklist can help reduce many errors, including that of wrong-site surgery. Treasure Coast Center for surgery shared their patient safety checklist in the case study beginning on page 78.

Table 4-4. Emergency Response in the Operating Room

Responding to a Surgical Wound Fire
1. Shut down medical gases.
2. Pour saline into the surgical site (unless it is an alcohol-fueled fire).
3. Remove the surgical drapes to the floor, along with any material that may have been burning.
4. Search for and extinguish any additional flames.
5. If the room contains smoke, determine whether it is necessary to evacuate.
6. Save all materials for later investigation (root cause analysis, as covered in Chapter 5, can provide a means of determining areas for improvement in preparedness for the future).

Responding to a Patient Airway Fire
1. Disconnect the breathing circuit from the tracheal tube.
2. Remove the tracheal tube and have another surgical team member extinguish it.
3. Remove any other segments of burned tube, such as any cuff protective devices, that may remain in the area.
4. Reestablish the airway and resume ventilating with air until certain nothing is left burning in the airway.
5. Examine airway for extent of damage.
6. Save all materials for later investigation.

Source: The Joint Commission: *Safety in the Operating Room.* Oakbrook Terrace, IL: Joint Commission Resources, 2006.

TOOL: Checklists

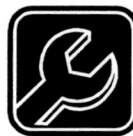

A number of excellent tools are available for use as a surgical checklist. One is the tool developed by Treasure Coast Center for Surgery, in Stuart, Florida (see Figure 4-5, page 80, later in this chapter).

Marking the Operative Site

Joint Commission Universal Protocol requirements call for designating a method of marking the surgical site, including ensuring that the type of mark is unambiguous and is used consistently throughout the organization. The procedure site should be marked by a licensed independent practitioner or other provider who is privileged or permitted by the organization to perform the intended surgical or nonsurgical invasive procedure. This individual will be involved directly in the procedure and will be present at the time the procedure is performed.

Table 4-5. What Is a Surgical Site Infection (SSI)?

Type of Infection	Time Frame	Tissue Involved	Signs and Symptoms
Superficial incisional infection	Develops within 30 days after the surgical procedure	Skin or subcutaneous tissue of the incision	■ Purulent drainage or organisms isolated from an aseptically obtained culture from the area ■ One sign and symptom of infection, such as pain or tenderness, localized swelling, redness, or heat ■ Superficial incision opened by the surgeon
Deep incisional infection	Develops within 30 days after the procedure or within one year of an implant placement	Deep soft tissues of the incision	■ Purulent drainage from the deep incision but not from the organ or space component of the surgery ■ Deep incision dehisced or opened by a surgeon when patient has fever, localized pain, or tenderness ■ An abscess or other evidence of infection found ■ Deep incisional SSI diagnosed by a surgeon or attending physician
Infection of the organ or space	Develops within 30 days after surgery or within one year if an implant is in place.	Any part of the anatomy (other than the incision) that was opened or manipulated during surgery	■ Purulent drainage from a drain placed into the organ or space ■ Organisms isolated from a culture of fluid or tissue in the organ/space ■ An abscess or other evidence of infection ■ Surgeon or attending physician diagnosed an organ/space SSI

Source: Odom-Forren J.: Preventing surgical site infections. *Nursing* 36:58–63, Jun. 2006.

Again, the patient is your best touchstone. Patient involvement is a critical component in efforts to minimize wrong-site, wrong-side surgeries. Also, do not assume that you have been given accurate information. Double-check information and materials at every step of the procedure. Just because a diagnosis is listed in the patient's record doesn't mean it is correct. Even the diagnosis needs a double check, including verifying imaging. Adverse events are rarely due to a single error, but instead result from a series of errors. Lastly, encourage all staff to "speak up" when their intuition or data tell them something is wrong.[19]

For procedures involving right/left distinction, multiple structures (such as fingers and toes), or multiple levels (as in spinal procedures), the intended site must be marked in such a way that the mark will be visible after the patient has been prepped and draped.

Effective Time-Outs

The time-out is conducted prior to starting the procedure and, ideally, prior to introducing the anesthesia process. Active communication among all members of the surgical/procedure team should be consistently initiated by a designated member of the team. Do not begin the procedure until providers ask all their questions and voice their concerns. Only when these concerns are resolved is working in a "fail-safe" mode facilitated.

It might seem optimal to perform a time-out just before beginning the surgical incision or commencing the procedure, but this may not always be possible due to logistical constraints related to the procedure or patients' needs, as well as concerns regarding performing incorrect anesthesia procedures. Each organization should define in which circumstances the time-out is required prior to anesthesia or when it is preferable to

---

Sidebar 4-2. Preventive Practices for Reducing Surgical Site Infections

- *Preoperative preparation of the patient.* This includes assessing the patient so that all infections remote from the surgical site can be treated before the procedure is performed. Ideally, elective procedures should be postponed until any infection has been resolved.
- *Antimicrobial prophylaxis* where appropriate (only when indicated and selected based on efficacy against the most common pathogens associated with surgical site infections [SSIs] for a specific procedure).
  —Standardize processes according to the range of procedures performed at your setting and to remove the necessity of writing a unique antibiotic order for every patient. This can help prevent prescription error or omission. The protocol should ensure that when the patient has allergies, or when a physician should be contacted for a different order, an appropriate substitution can be made easily.* The Surgical Care Improvement Project (SCIP; *see* Chapter 5, "Infection Prevention and Control") provides resources and guidance on the use of prophylactic antibiotics.
  —Document in a standardized place the dose given and the time of incision. Research shows that the timing of the first dose of prophylaxis plays a crucial role in the risk for SSIs.* Ideally the first dose is given 30–60 minutes before the incision is made. The antibiotic dose should be adjusted for the patient's actual (not estimated) weight.
  —Determine a policy in your organization for the discontinuation of antibiotic use. Protocols and standard order sets can help ensure that antibiotics are stopped at the appropriate time.
  —Provide supplemental oxygen during surgery, if warranted. Maintaining high levels of inspired oxygen can help reduce SSIs.*
- *Asepsis and proper surgical technique.* Asepsis is important for procedures in which intravascular devices are placed, spinal or epidural anesthesia catheters are placed, or intravenous medications are dispensed or administered. Perform meticulous hand hygiene.
  —Create policies for proper hair removal, glycemic control, and warming patients.
  —Keep hair removal to an absolute minimum. Research shows a lower rate of infection when patients do not have hair removed.* Although it has been known for decades that shaving patients prior to surgery increases risk of infections, some people are reluctant to change how they were originally trained. Make it policy to use clippers rather than razors, and provide proper training in using clippers. Instruct patients not to shave near the surgical site prior to arriving at the AHC setting for surgery, and to shower or bathe prior to surgery using antiseptic soap.†
  —Ensure glycemic control. Higher blood sugar levels have been shown to increase the risk of SSIs.* Postoperatively, the patient's glucose levels can be remaintained.
  —Maintain patient temperature so that oxygen-rich blood flowing to the incision site promotes faster healing. Hypothermia has been shown to increase risk of SSIs. Use a combination of blankets, forced-air patient warming systems, warmed intravenous (IV) fluids, or slightly elevated room temperatures.* Monitor the patient's temperature in the operating room (OR) and recovery area. A temporal scanner thermometer is easy to use and may be more accurate than other types of thermometers. Keep patients covered until just before the surgical site must be exposed. Consider having them wear a hat and booties during surgery.† Also expose a minimal area while prepping the patient.
- *Postoperative incision care.* The Centers for Disease Control and Prevention guidelines recommend protecting surgical sites with sterile dressing for 24 to 48 hours after closing the incision "primarily." When a dressing must be changed, and if this must involve the patient and/or family, thorough education is essential. Teach patients how to spot signs and symptoms of infection, and give them a contact number to call if a problem arises.
- *Surveillance.* Postoperative and postdischarge surveillance can help spot trends in, among other areas, types of infection, populations most affected, and most problematic procedures. Ensure proper data collection with agreement on standardized definitions. This involves limiting interpretation about what constitutes an SSI to specified criteria.

* The Joint Commission: *Safety in the Operating Room.* Oakbrook Terrace, IL: Joint Commission Resources, 2006.
† Odom-Forren J.: Preventing surgical site infections. *Nursing* 36:58–63, Jun. 2006.

---

conduct a time-out immediately before beginning the procedure or making the initial incision.

Standardization

The most effective way to keep on point with the day's surgical schedule and still protect patient safety is to standardize, standardize, standardize. Keep an eye out for all ways that systems can be made into routines, and staff can be trained to adhere to those routines and standards. However, remember that each patient is an individual and must be treated as such. Forms can be standard, people are not.

Sidebar 4-3. Steps in the Universal Protocol to Prevent Wrong-Site, Wrong Procedure, and Wrong Person Surgery™

The Joint Commission is currently reviewing the content of the Universal Protocol. As of this writing, these steps include the following:

Conduct a preprocedure verification process.
The preprocedure verification is an ongoing process of information gathering and verification, beginning with the decision to perform a procedure, continuing through all settings and interventions involved in the preprocedure preparation of the [patient], up to and including the time-out just before the start of the procedure.

Mark the procedure site.
Marking the procedure site allows staff to identify without ambiguity the intended site for the procedure.

Perform a time-out immediately prior to starting procedures.
The purpose of the time-out immediately before starting the procedure is to conduct a final assessment that the correct [patient], site, positioning, and procedure are identified and that, as applicable, all relevant documents, related information, and necessary equipment are available. The time-out is consistently initiated by a designated member of the team and includes active communication among all relevant members of the procedure team. It is conducted in a standardized fail-safe mode (that is, the procedure is not started until all questions or concerns are resolved).

Source: The Joint Commission.

As mentioned previously in this chapter, an example of standardization that sped up flow was the administration of antibiotic prophylaxis, which should be given to the patient no later than 60 minutes before the first incision is made to prevent SSIs.[20] At one organization in Middlebury, Vermont, it was observed that nurses were taking vital signs, checking patient history, and handling other responsibilities before giving the patient the antibiotic. This slowed down scheduling in the OR as the day proceeded. To remedy the slowdown, surgical teams specified the order in which tasks were accomplished, which includes having nurses begin administering prophylaxis before completing their other tasks.

References

1. ECRI Institute and Institute for Safe Medication Practices: Obstructive sleep apnea may block the path to a positive postoperative outcome. *PA-PSRS Patient Safety Advisory* 4:91, Sep. 2007.

2. The Joint Commission: *Safety in the Operating Room.* Oakbrook Terrace, IL: Joint Commission Resources, 2006.

3. Desai M.S.: Office-based anesthesia: New frontiers, better outcomes, and emphasis on safety. *Curr Opin Anaesthesiol* 21:699–703, Dec. 2008.

4. Gaca A.M., Lerner C.B., Frush D.P.: The radiology perspective: Needs and tools for management of life-threatening events. *Pediatr Radiol* 38(suppl. 4):S714–S719, Nov. 2008.

5. Gaca A.M., et al.: Enhancing pediatric safety: Using simulation to assess radiology resident preparedness for anaphylaxis from intravenous contrast media. *Radiology* 245:236–244, Oct. 2007.

6. Children's Hospital and Health System Inc: *Patient Care Policy and Procedure: Procedural Sedation.* 2007. http://www.chw.org/staff/FVProceduralSedation.doc (accessed Mar. 6, 2009).

7. Institute for Safe Medication Practices, Health Research and Educational Trust, and Medical Group Management Association: *The Physician Practice Patient Safety Assessment.* 2005. http://www.coloradopatientsafety.org/PPPSAcompleteMay06.pdf (accessed Feb. 20, 2009).

8. Hennepin County Medical Center: *Care of Patients Undergoing Moderate and Deep Procedural Sedation.* http://www.hcmc.org/education/residency/ documents/proceduralsedation.pdf (accessed Mar. 6, 2009).

9. Malignant Hyperthermia Association of the United States: *MHAUS Guidelines. Testing for Malignant Hyperthermia (MH) Susceptibility: How do I counsel my patients?* http://medical.mhaus.org/NonFB/Slideshow_eng/SlideShow_ENG_files/frame.htm (accessed Feb. 27, 2009).

10. Dixon B.A., O'Donnell J.M.: Is your patient susceptible to malignant hyperthermia? *Nursing* 36:26–27, Dec. 2006.

11. Klein B.R., Ginsburg E.: *Ambulatory Surgical Centers and Emergency Power: Why? What? And for How Long?* Sep. 1, 2008. http://ecmweb.com/design_engineering/electric_ambulatory_surgical_centers/ (accessed Mar. 9, 2009).

12. Salmon L.: Fire in the OR—Prevention and preparedness. *AORN J* 80:41–54, Jul. 2004.

13. Bellino J.V.: Operating room fire safety. *J Healthc Prot Manage* 23(1):115–124, 2007.

14. Caplan R.A., et al.: Practice advisory for the prevention and management of operating room fires. *Anesthesiology* 108:786–801, May 2008.

15. University of Illinois at Chicago: *Fire Safety Instructions.* 2009. http://www.uic.edu/depts/envh/HSS/Fire.html (accessed Mar. 8, 2009).

16. The Joint Commission: *Engaging Physicians in Patient Safety: A Handbook for Leaders.* Oakbrook Terrace, IL: Joint Commission Resources, 2006.

17. MedQIC: *Surgical Care Improvement Project. Making Surgery Safer Project Overview.* http://www.qualitynet.org/dcs/ContentServer?pagename=Medqic/MQPage/Homepage (accessed Mar. 1, 2009).

18. Mangram A.J., et al.: Guideline for prevention of surgical site infection, 1999. Hospital Infection Control Practices Advisory Committee. *Infect Control Hosp Epidemiol* 20:250–278, Apr. 1999.

19. AHC Media. Wrong-site surgery: We're not doing all that we can. *Healthcare Benchmarks and Quality Improvement* 15:49–60, Jun. 2008.

20. Beauregard A., Rogers M., Spry C.: Surgical site infection rate drops to zero in months. *Same-Day Surgery* 65–67, Jun. 1, 2006.

Case Study: Malignant Hyperthermia

CASE STUDY AT A GLANCE

Organization: Malignant Hyperthermia Association of the United States (MHAUS); Emory Healthcare, Atlanta; and the Surgical Center of York, York, Pennsylvania.

Setting: National nongovernmental organization (MHAUS), an academic anesthesiology department, and an ambulatory surgery center (ASC)

Patient safety topic: Development and adoption of a procedure manual for the treatment of malignant hyperthermia (MH)

Accomplishment: The program improved the awareness, efficiency, and response time for cases of MH. This was accomplished by the use of a new Checklist and Worksheet Tool, organization of the anesthesiology and operating room (OR) teams, and the creation of a stocked MH cart.

The Organization

The Surgical Center of York, a multispecialty ASC in York, Pennsylvania, adopted for its use the Malignant Hyperthermia Procedure Manual developed by a member of the Department of Anesthesiology at Emory Healthcare in Atlanta, and MHAUS.

The Surgical Center of York performs approximately 2,400 procedures a year ranging from otolaryngology, ophthalmology, and orthopedics as well as gynecologic surgery, general surgery, and podiatry. The patient age ranges from 6 months to more than 95 years old. The safety culture starts at the top.

Project Beginnings

Project Name and Goals

The Malignant Hyperthermia Procedure Manual was developed to provide a rapid response plan to implement recommended therapies from MHAUS quickly and efficiently using available OR personnel, the checklist approach, and a method of organizing supplies and treatment medications into an MH cart.

Needs Identification and Baseline Measures

MH is a rapidly progressive hypermetabolic response that a patient may experience unexpectedly when exposed to certain anesthetic agents. There may be no knowledge of patient susceptibility, and the condition may occur in any setting in which these triggering agents are used. MH is a potentially lethal problem that leads to electrolyte abnormalities and mixed respiratory/metabolic acidosis with rapid progression to cardiovascular collapse if untreated. Delay in treatment leads to multisystem organ failure such as cerebral edema, diffuse intravascular coagulapathy, and renal failure. Successful treatment of MH depends on early recognition of signs and symptoms and rapid treatment. Minutes matter and multiple tasks need to be accomplished rapidly.

Colleagues of the members of the Procedure Manual development team shared anecdotal reports of the complex treatment of this rare syndrome. Those experienced in the treatment of a patient with MH emphasized the rapid onset and progression of the patient to an unstable situation. They universally affirmed the need for an easy-to-follow, organizational team response plan to aid with efficiency in the treatment of MH.

After reviewing the concurrent steps (as recommended by MHAUS), and considering the immediacy needed to institute those steps in the treatment of MH, the developer of the Procedure Manual conducted a test using an unannounced drill for a mock episode of MH. She found that the problem was a coordination-response-team issue that could be improved. This anesthesiologist and her team set forth to develop an organized, easy-to-follow approach to coordinate the staff who would be responding to an episode of MH.

Subsequent mock MH episodes were then used to develop the response plan. The team realized that the complex treatment recommendations could be completed efficiently and in a timely manner by centralizing supplies on a cart and organizing the available OR staff with a concise set of worksheets in a checklist format. The MHAUS team, along with the

Case Study: Malignant Hyperthermia (continued)

Emory team, further refined the response plan to make it more universally applicable to other centers.

At the Surgical Center of York, MH is given a high level of importance because this ASC is located in South Central Pennsylvania, which has a higher incidence of MH compared with other areas. This is due to the fact that families do not often spread out to other regions of the country; therefore the hereditary factors are more critical.

Team Members and Roles

The concept of worksheets and assigned tasks to implement the MHAUS treatment recommendations was developed for the Grady Health System, Atlanta, by Darlene Mashman, M.D., an assistant professor of anesthesiology at Emory. She conducted mock drills in developing the response plan and assigned response team roles. She assisted another team member who took responsibility for stocking the MH cart with medications and supplies recommended by MHAUS.

The response plan was presented at the 1996 American Society of Anesthesiologists Annual Meeting as a scientific exhibit where the president of MHAUS invited the Emory team to work with the staff at MHAUS to create the Procedure Manual. The MHAUS team, along with the Emory team, further worked on the response plan to allow it to be adaptable to other centers. MHAUS received an unrestricted educational grant from a pharmaceutical company to develop the manual. Others were involved in designing and producing the manual's illustrations, and developing and producing a mock drill video and the videotape for distribution.

At the Surgical Center of York, the team leader was the clinical services manager, who was in charge of the adoption of the manual for her ASC. This ASC's patient safety team reports to the quality council, which then reports to the board of directors.

Project Activity
Project Steps
The development team identified the need for an easy-to-implement response tool for rapid treatment of a complex syndrome and developed a way to improve team organization using the concept of worksheets similar to checklists of the airline industry. A cart containing the equipment and supplies as well as treatment medications was produced using MHAUS recommendations. Mock MH drills were conducted to test usefulness of the response plan. OR staff were asked for input regarding ease of use. Timing of treatment and the observed organization of the responders to the drills were assessed.

The Tools Used
Tools used for the response plan include the Procedure Manual describing the response plan in detail, a flow sheet, the worksheets, signs reminding staff of supplies location and procedure (which may be posted in area such as the break room), a video of the response plan being used during a mock drill, and mock drill performance sheets (to track progress). The ASC used the supplies guide to make an MH cart and checklist for that cart. The supply list was used to improve the current list of medications and supplies. The drill guide was used as a template for various other drill types that the organization runs, such as pandemic, cardiac, fire, and weather drills.

Old Process/Plan vs. New
Previously, awareness was "spotty" and materials and supplies to treat MH were in various locations. In the new procedure, the MH cart centralized materials and supplies and includes the checklist worksheet, which directs responders to supplies that cannot be contained on the cart (such as ice or insulin). This worksheet is shown in Figure 4-3, page 74.

Previously, verbal communication was needed to direct OR staff during a time of crisis. Communication was improved using checklists handed out from the MH cart to OR staff by the anes-

(continued on page 74)

Case Study: Malignant Hyperthermia (continued)

Figure 4-3. Circulator/OR Charge Nurse Worksheet for an MH Event in the Operating Room

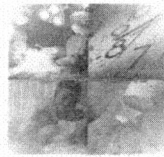

MALIGNANT HYPERTHERMIA
PROCEDURE MANUAL

Circulator/OR Charge Nurse Worksheet
Malignant Hyperthermia Event in the OR

Procedures for a Malignant Hyperthermia Crisis

√ when completed

_____ 1) Announce event initiating response protocol.

"Attention All Personnel: Malignant Hyperthermia in OR # _____."

"Malignant Hyperthermia cart/kit to OR # _____, STAT."

_____ 2) Assist ATA/ORNA in obtaining supplies.

_____ 3) Assist in mixing Dantrolene.

_____ 4) Prepare and place ice packs to groin and axilla.

_____ 5) Place the foley catheter
- send urine sample for myoglobin
- lavage bladder with cold saline if needed

_____ 6) Coordinate/assist nursing team and ensure all tasks are completed.

AFTER PATIENT IS STABLE:

_____ 1) Help transport patient to PACU.

_____ 2) Assure restocking of anesthesia and nursing supplies on MH cart/kit and refrigerator.

_____ 3) Ensure MH cart/kit has been returned to designated location.

Copyright © 2001, Malignant Hyperthermia Association of the US   17

The task checklists efficiently and clearly help the OR staff to communicate during a time of crisis.

Source: Malignant Hyperthermia Association of the United States, Procedure Manual.

Case Study: Malignant Hyperthermia (continued)

Figure 4-4. Event Drill Worksheet

The event drill worksheet is the record keeping item for a mock drill, and is used to check progress from drill to drill.

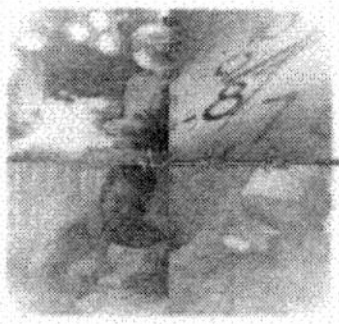

MALIGNANT HYPERTHERMIA
PROCEDURE MANUAL

Malignant Hyperthermia
Event Drill

Date

Drill Location (OR #)

Conducted by

Attending Anesthesiologist

Arrival of Items

Malignant Hyperthermia Cart/Kit

Chilled 1000 ml normal saline bags for IV infusion

Bags of cold normal saline for irrigation

3000 ml saline bags for bladder and NG irrigation

Ice

Regular insulin 100 units/ml

Arrival Times

Responders

Surgeon

Anesthetist/Anesthesiologist

Circulator/OR Charge Nurse

PACU Charge Nurse

Scrub Nurse/OR Tech

ATA/ORNA

Organization of Team: Poor   Fair   Good   Excellent

Comments/Areas of Improvement:

20

Timing of treatment and the observed organization of the responders to the drills are assessed via the Event Drill form.

Source: Malignant Hyperthermia Association of the United States, Procedure Manual.

(continued on page 76)

Case Study: Malignant Hyperthermia (continued)

thesiologist. Efficiency and organization were improved. In the old process, missing a step was a risk. The checklist of tasks minimized this risk. In addition, before the development and use of the manual, coordinating responders was challenging. Responders now aid the OR team quickly and efficiently by following the task lists.

Also, the old process was simply to rely on information gathered from articles and experience. For instance, the old process to reconstitute the Dantrium was to use 3,000 mL bags of sterile water and 60 mL syringes with 18 gauge needles and a lot of manpower. This took several people and was very time consuming. Using the process described in the Malignant Hyperthermia Procedure Manual simplified this a great deal. The procedure is now closed and more sterile. Because the nurse does not have to use a needle, unnecessary needlesticks are prevented, and thus this is a much safer procedure.

Staff Training and Education

On receiving the new Procedure Manual, ASC management studied it and then presented it to the staff. The Procedure Manual did not need to be adapted. It was very explicit and easy to follow. The video, along with the information, provided consistent information across the entire system. After everyone was familiar with this information a surprise drill was called. This put into process everyone ranging from anesthesia to nurses to receptionists and helped the team evaluate the information learned and the technique used.

An educational in-service is needed at least one time per year to educate staff about MH and to demonstrate the response plan. Periodic drills test the team in the use of the plan, test the system for preparedness in the treatment of MH, and demonstrate the need for further staff education.

The Outcome
Measurable Outcomes
Measurable outcomes are documented by increased awareness of MH and improved response times. This is shown by documentation on the event drill form, presented in Figure 4-4, page 75. This form shows the date of drill and arrival times of the various items needed for the treatment of a patient experiencing MH. It documents who responded and scores the organization of the team as poor, fair, good, or excellent and gives an area for comments.

Lessons Learned

The ASC staff is composed of many part-time people. It was a challenge to communicate who would be in charge of different responsibilities pertaining to the drill. (After the initial orientation to the manual and practice drill, the ASC continues to stage one mock drill each year.) The team put in place a white board listing the different responsibilities such as ice, MH cart, and so forth, and each day a staff name is written there. It is everyone's responsibility to read that board. One person is responsible for assigning these names. The names are also consistent with the area in which the person is working. For example, a front desk receptionist is always in charge of ice. A recovery room staff member is in charge of the cart. Being in charge of the cart also entails checking it each month for outdates and supply needs. For ASC staff, mixing the Dantrium was found to be easier than expected. The diagram included in the manual simplified the mixing instructions. It is also easier to follow a visual instruction during a time of emergency than reading an explanation.

One big lesson learned was how to provide education to all staff because of the busy ongoing schedule maintained at this ASC. It can be difficult to get everyone's attention on the issues. The training video provided a means to educate everyone with consistent information. The drill guide then helped them implement a drill. After the practice drill, they realized they do not draw blood for lab tests very often. The type of tube and equipment is not familiar to everyone due to this low level of use. The staff have now taken responsibility to create a kit with exactly the correct lab tube, lab slips, and other equipment necessary to draw

Case Study: Malignant Hyperthermia (continued)

blood without wasting time researching which tube they want and where to get it. The lab requests are completed ahead of time so they are ready to send immediately with the vials. The event drill worksheet made documentation of the drill easy and concise.

Perhaps the most critical issue related to their success concerned recognizing that providing staff education regarding MH and having a ready response plan are critical, and performing a mock drill to confirm that the plan works for a specific institution and its staff is very important. The Clinical Services Manager reports: "In my 30 years of nursing I have never seen a case of MH. It is difficult to teach and retain information regarding something you have never experienced. This manual provided an easy, efficient method of teaching. It also provides education material that will be used over and over again."

Case Study: Safety Checklist

CASE STUDY AT A GLANCE

Organization: Treasure Coast Center for Surgery, Stuart, Florida

Setting: Ambulatory surgery center

Patient safety topic: Use of an original patient safety checklist

Accomplishment: The Center has experienced no near misses or adverse events since initiating the use of this list.

The Organization

Treasure Coast Center for Surgery is a multispecialty ambulatory surgery center (ASC) in Stuart, Florida. Specialties represented include ophthalmology, orthopedics, spine, podiatry, pain management, and GI endoscopy. They have also just recruited two new specialties, gynecology and urology. Meridian Surgical Partners, headquartered in Brentwood, Tennessee, is the management company and majority owner of the facility. Treasure Coast has taken care of patients ranging in age from young adults to the elderly.

Treasure Coast's leadership and administration includes a vice president of operations, a clinical administrator/registered nurse (R.N.), a business office manager, and a materials management director.

Project Beginnings

Project Name and Goals

The project was first presented in Nashville at the annual conference of the Ambulatory Surgery Center Association (ASCA). The team leader used the metaphor of a model plane, per the aviation industry, to compare the use of the handoff report checklist with the preflight checklist used for aviation safety:

Do your preflight handoff report checklist in preparation for take off: Time out for safety; improve care for a safe landing.

The project was officially begun in March 2009.

Needs Identification and Baseline Measures

A couple of near misses were noted by nursing. The near misses regarded wrong-site surgeries. These close-call events were documented in the log that the staff maintain in the reception area of the Center for just this purpose. When nursing read of these occasions, it prompted them to develop a new checklist tool (described below).

Team Members and Roles

The team consisted of the clinical administrator/R.N. (Team Leader), the facility's medical director, the full-time anesthesiologist, and two nurses: an operating room (OR) nurse and a preoperative/preoperative anesthetic care nurse.

Project Activity

Project Steps

After these near misses were noted by nursing, the team leader conducted research to review the criteria that The Joint Commission and other safety organizations were looking for in a checklist. The team compared the existing checklist tool with others viewed on the Internet and increased their knowledge in this area. The checklist tool that had been used was then modified accordingly.

The team then met to discuss how to design the tool to involve all three areas of the facility: preoperative care, the OR, and the recovery department. They wanted to make sure to improve communication among the three areas, because the flow process of the checklist ensures that the preoperative nurse is handing off a report to the OR nurse, and the OR nurse is handing off a report to the recovery room nurse. The method of communication is now similar to that of the SBAR technique, a formalized method of communication between health care providers. (SBAR denotes Situation, Background, Assessment, Recommendation.) That is, communication needed to be accurate and succinct, and specific relevant issues and concerns needed to be highlighted in each communication.

Case Study: Safety Checklist (continued)

The Tools Used

The checklist is a tool for effective team communication, safe surgery, efficient teamwork, and prevention of wrong-site surgery. This checklist tool is presented in Figure 4-5, page 80.

Old Process/Plan vs. New

In the old process, the ASC also employed a checklist, but that worksheet involved only the OR nurse. The OR nurse was the only person who would fill it out and even look at it before it was completed. The OR nurse would ensure that the patient was identified, that the physician had marked the surgical site, and that a time-out was done; it was simply a "one person show" and did not involve any other team members. Because no double checks were performed, this method did not allow a means of catching errors or bringing up problems and concerns for all to address before a procedure was begun.

In the new process, the checklist tool necessitates staff confirming that everything in the patient's chart matches everything in the medical record. It also requires staff to match that information with information in the surgical schedule and with the patient's response. Staff are finding it to be a terrific means of engaging different departments in effectively communicating with each other about patient care.

One aspect that was newly introduced to the modified checklist tool was on-time antibiotic administration, recommended by The Joint Commission and other quality and safety organizations. Antibiotics are now administered within one hour prior to initiating a surgical procedure.

Staff Training and Education

To get the staff engaged, the team held a meeting the morning the new tool was to begin being used. The team leader explained it would replace the preexisting checklist, why they were changing it, and how it would improve communication and make surgery safer and more efficient. Staff were already somewhat familiar with the new tool as it was being developed, but they hadn't been officially in-serviced to use it. Therefore, at the launch of the checklist on that first day, this meeting served as a training session.

The ASC has 30 employees. Nursing alone was involved in this meeting because the nurses are the ones who document on the tool. However, where a team approach was involved—that is, in conducting a time-out and ensuring that correct implants and any special equipment were available—the entire team recognized that this was a new tool, and the surgeon and the OR technician became fully involved in answering to their respective areas of responsibility when filling out the tool preprocedure.

On the first day the new checklist was used, after the meeting adjourned, the nursing staff were a bit uncertain about using this new tool, and therefore they were a bit resistant. Some items are not applicable to all surgeries, and they felt it would take more time to fill out the new document. This was also true in the case of diagnostic laboratory results, where there were now more areas to document. To resolve this problem, the team added "NA" (not applicable) boxes to the list to make it easier for the nurses to quickly, but carefully, document all areas. This helped encourage the nurses to use the checklist.

The process evolved and was incorporated smoothly. The surgeons were all on board because they had been fully trained in the necessity of using such a checklist to promote patient safety. As mentioned, the biggest obstacle of the project was introducing the new form to the nurses, because they were not happy to grapple with what they felt to be additional tasks of paperwork. However, after the team explained the need for and importance of using the new tool, the nurses understood and took it on more enthusiastically.

The Outcome
Measurable Outcomes
Although not measurable so far, the staff believe that

(continued on page 80)

Case Study: Safety Checklist (continued)

Figure 4-5. Checklist for Patient Handoffs to Surgery

TREASURE COAST CENTER FOR SURGERY

HANDOFF REPORT CHECKLIST	Pre-Op Initials	OR Initials	OR Initials	PACU Initials
Patient Verification / Patient Identified *(Patient states name & date of birth, information verified on ID band)*				
Patient's statement of correct Procedure/Side/Site matches Informed Consent				
Physician's Informed Consent/Orders/History & Physical/ Surgical Schedule/Surgeon's Notes are consistent with patient response.				
If any discrepancy, Stop until resolved!!!	STOP	STOP	STOP	STOP
Consent for Procedure(s) signed and witnessed				
Consent for Anesthesia signed and witnessed ☐ **NA** *(for local cases only)*				
Allergies Verified ☐ **NKA**				
Medical Clearance on chart ☐ **NA**				
Diagnostic Labs on chart: ☐ **NA**				
CBC				
SMA				
PT/PTT ☐ **NA**				
U/A ☐ **NA**				
EKG ☐ **NA**				
CXR ☐ **NA**				
On Time IV Antibiotic Administration *(initiated within 1 hour prior to procedure, with the exception of vancomycin or fluoroquinolones, delivery should be within 2 hours prior to procedure)*				
Surgical Site is marked/verified by the Physician performing the surgery/procedure with his/ her initials				
Pertinent Radiological Studies are available *(e.g. X-rays)* ☐ **NA**				
ALL correct implants and any special equipment needed is present and functional.				
Time Out performed & confirmed by Entire Team immediately prior to the start of the procedure.				
Complete Handoff Report given to RN				
Transferred via: A- *Ambulatory* **S-** *Stretcher* **W-** *Wheelchair*				

INITIALS	NURSE SIGNATURE	
		Patient ID

The handoff report checklist now facilitates better communication and teamwork.

Source: Treasure Coast Center for Surgery.

Case Study: Safety Checklist (continued)

communication and teamwork have improved appreciably. No near misses or errors have occurred thus far since beginning use of the checklist two months ago.

This project has made the nurses from other departments in the ASC (preoperative care, the OR, and the recovery department) aware of the importance of having a handoff tool, the importance of knowing and having the correct implants and equipment ready, and knowing about and being aware of on-time antibiotic administration. They now view this as a team effort, requiring a team approach between nurses and among staff and providers. They recognize that responsibility for this method and for patient safety as a whole should not just be delegated to one person alone.

The team intends to follow up in six months to review and assess whether anything needs to be added to, modified, or deleted from the checklist. They also intend to study whether the form is being used in the way and with the regularity with which it was intended, and to recruit staff comments and contributions.

Lessons Learned

Every year the organization leaders attend the ASCA conference. At each conference all the facilities owned by Meridian present a poster project, and Meridian sponsors a contest for the best poster project. These presentations address patient safety and sharing what they've learned and improved at their ASC. The team presented this project at this year's meeting.

Treasure Coast's staff and patients read regularly in both the scientific literature and the lay press about the issues related to patient safety, particularly as they pertain to surgery. The team reports that because they read so many reports about errors and problems that occur, and because they recognize they are all human and humans do make errors, they now understand that introducing patient safety initiatives and introducing a new culture that values patient safety is paramount. Public awareness has bolstered commitment to take on initiatives of this sort. Openness with nursing, surgeons, anesthesia, and technicians is now more valued and improved at this organization.

In terms of how this culture affects reporting occurrences and close calls, the team believes that the facility's nursing staff feel more supported in reporting mistakes and close calls (which they do in an occurrence report, as seen in Figure 4-6, page 82). The nurses are the number one patient advocates. They are speaking up to say, "These types of errors can't happen here." There have been no obstacles or further challenges in implementing this tool. The team is currently collecting data and discussing what new tool can best monitor that the tool is continually used properly and any problems or events are documented in the Center's occurrence report.

(continued on page 82)

Case Study: Safety Checklist (continued)

Figure 4-6. Occurrence Report

Report
Treasure Coast Center for Surgery (TCCFS)

The report serves as a loss control for Risk Management and Quality Improvement Analysis and for the use by the facility's attorneys in anticipation of litigation. The person most closely involved or the person discovering the must complete this form as soon as possible. Complete entire form.

Patient Label Or Employee/Visitor/Other Name	Age	Sex [ ]M [ ]F	Date of Incident
	Date of Service		| |- | |- | | |
			Time of Incident
	Medical Record #		

Admitting Diagnosis: _____

Procedure: _____
Please check appropriate information:
1. **Identification:**
   [] Patient   [] Visitor   [] Employee   [] Other _____

Address _____ **Telephone #** _____

2. **Location:**
   [] Business Office [] Pre-op Area [] O.R. [] PACU [] Procedure Room [] Other _____

3. **Brief Objective Description** (factual information only – include VS, X-Rays, Labs, follow-up care, etc.)
   _____
   _____
   _____
   _____
   _____
   _____

4. If this was a medication reaction, did incident meet criteria for reporting to the FDA?
   [ ]Yes [ ]No [ ] N/A

5. If the incident involved equipment, write the Equipment I.D. # and present location [ ] N/A.
   _____

6. Is this incident reportable under the Safe Medical Devices Act? [ ]Yes [ ]No [ ]N/A

7. **Physician Notified** _____ Date & Time _____
   Medical Tx. Recommended _____ [ ] None
8. **Treatment given by:** [ ]Physician _____ [ ]E.D. _____ [ ]Refused
9. **Persons Involved Including Witnesses**   **Indicate Where Person Can Be Located**
   _____   [ ] TCCFS or _____
   _____   [ ] TCCFS or _____
   _____   [ ] TCCFS or _____

| Person Completing Report (Name Printed <u>and</u> Title) | Signature | Date and Time |
| Risk Manager/ Designee Notified [ ] Yes [ ] No | Date _____ | Time _____ |

CONFIDENTIAL – NOT A PART OF A PATIENT'S MEDICAL RECORD- DO NOT COPY

An occurrence report includes all pertinent information of an error or close call.

Source: Treasure Coast Center for Surgery.

Chapter 5

INFECTION PREVENTION AND CONTROL

The spread of infection is more in the news today than ever before. The threat of bioterrorism, the resistance of common pathogens to antibiotics, and an overall increase in infectious diseases such as HIV and hepatitis have all increased public awareness of infection prevention and control (IC). Health care–associated infections (HAIs) remain a serious problem in health care.[1] The Centers for Medicare & Medicaid Services (CMS) has revised Conditions for Coverage (CfC) and added requirements in the IC arena, which has spurred a major focus on IC for ambulatory providers. In CfC 416.51, an ambulatory surgery center (ASC) must maintain an IC program that minimizes infections and communicable diseases. The facility must provide a functional and sanitary environment for the provision of surgical services by adhering to professionally acceptable standards of practice, and the infection prevention program must include documentation that the ASC has considered, selected, and implemented nationally recognized IC guidelines, such as those issued by the Centers for Disease Control and Prevention (CDC). Other issues that point to the need for caution with regard to IC in AHC include sterilization processes (*see* Chapter 6, "Environment and Equipment"), dialysis patient care, use of multidose solutions, cross contamination of instruments, and lack of airborne infection isolation rooms.[2]

Reducing the risk and preventing the spread of infection is a safety priority and requirement for all AHC organizations. Each AHC organization requires attention specific to its setting and population. For example, in hemodialysis units overall IC practices will include taking precautions to prevent transmission among patients, conducting routine serologic testing for hepatitis B (HBV) and hepatitis C (HCV), vaccinating susceptible patients against HBV, and isolating patients who test positive for HBV surface antigen. Risk reduction strategies for hemodialysis units include the following[2]:

- Adhering to strict aseptic technique during all dialysis procedures
- Adhering to strict procedures for using, disinfecting, and maintaining equipment
- Training staff members to understand the implications of deviating from established procedures
- Monitoring all procedures in which bacterial or chemical contamination can occur
- Conducting an effective patient education program that includes teaching patients and families how to play their part in preventing dialysis-related infections
- Routinely monitoring and following up with patients undergoing dialysis

A review of outbreak information collected in the decade between 1998 and 2008 revealed that 33 outbreaks of health care–associated HBV and HCV transmission occurred in ambulatory and other nonhospital settings. Of the 33 outbreaks, 12 occurred in ambulatory care clinics and 6 in hemodialysis centers, resulting in a total of 311 persons acquiring HBV or HCV infection in those settings. In each setting, the putative mechanism of infection was patient-to-patient transmission through failure of health care personnel to adhere to fundamental principles of IC and aseptic technique (for example, reusing syringes or lancing devices).[3] In another, well-known case, an endoscopy center in southern Nevada was linked to a 2008 outbreak of HCV, spurring an ongoing investigation (*see also* Chapter 4, "Surgical Safety").[4,5]

The good news is that these outbreaks are preventable. Standard precautions include injection safety and protocols for the use of shared equipment. These precautions apply in all settings that provide health care and represent the foundation of basic safe-care practices. A comprehensive preventive approach includes augmented viral hepatitis surveillance, education and training for health care providers in the appropriate practices and techniques, improved oversight, and more uniform regulation.

Additional safeguards can be installed with a patient-centric approach that includes the patient in planning for upcoming ambulatory surgical procedures. A document published by the Association for Professionals in Infection Control and Epidemiology, available online, includes useful information for discussion between patients and providers regarding proper infection control.[6] Topics covered include staff credentialing, cleaning and sterilization of the environment and equipment, antibiotic prophylaxis, site preparation and safe injection practices, maintaining normal body temperature, hand hygiene, using protective apparel, glucose control, and smoking cessation.

The Joint Commission has developed specific IC standards. These standards raise expectations for leadership and an IC program to run integrated, responsive processes throughout the organization and in coordination with other health care organizations. Leadership and managers must designate IC as a priority throughout the organization and allocate appropriate resources for a successful program.

For AHC settings, some particular issues are foremost in importance. Incorporating appropriate hand hygiene and cough etiquette are essential, as are disinfection and cleaning for equipment and the environment (see also Chapter 7, "Staff Education and Training"). Also important is tracking data associated with infection-related sentinel events. These topics are discussed below.

Hand Hygiene

Joint Commission requirements designate following the current hand hygiene guidelines recommended by the World Health Organization or the CDC. Tips modified from these CDC guidelines (the Clean Hands Save Lives campaign) are presented in Table 5-1, page 85.

When providers are managing an infected or draining wound, it is obvious that careful hand hygiene and gloving is of paramount importance. But normal, intact skin is also colonized by bacteria; the quantity depends on the area of the body. This means that activities such as taking a pulse or blood pressure, or lifting a patient, may still result in caregivers acquiring a significant volume of pathogens on their hands.[7]

Note that the CDC's "Vaccine Administration" Guidelines state that gloves are not required to be worn when administering vaccines unless the person administering the vaccine is likely to come into contact with potentially infectious body fluids or has open lesions on the hands. It is also important to remember that gloves cannot prevent needlestick injuries.[8]

Infections that are most often found in ambulatory care settings (and other health care settings) include surgical site infections (SSIs) (see section on the Surgical Care Improvement Project beginning on page 88 in this chapter and see Chapter 4, "Surgical Safety").

Despite the ongoing effort to improve compliance with good hand hygiene practices, compliance rates remain steady at about 25% to 50%.[7] Because patients come and go in ambulatory settings, staff may not make the connection between their poor hygiene practices and the onset of patient infection. This may be particularly true of staff in urgent care centers, for instance, which have a high volume of high-risk patients.

New waterless hand sanitizers are as effective as soap and water, and because sanitizers do not dry out hands, they are less likely to lead to dryness and subsequent skin cracks. Skin cracks can become reservoirs for pathogens, leading to infections among staff and transmission to others. Antimicrobial solutions have not proven beneficial as they may contribute to antibiotic resistance.

Although it is recommended that organizations teach patients to ask all caregivers whether they have washed their hands, this may be uncomfortable for many patients. Some organizations have identified creative solutions for this dilemma, with buttons patients can wear and point to, reminding them of proper hand hygiene and IC.

- -

TOOL: Visual Controls for Hand Hygiene

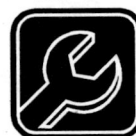

A number of useful visual controls are available to remind health care providers, as well as others in health care settings, to use proper hand hygiene when in contact with patients. Using visuals has been shown to improve compliance with hygiene guidelines. A few visual tools are provided as samples

Figure 5-1. Hand Hygiene Poster

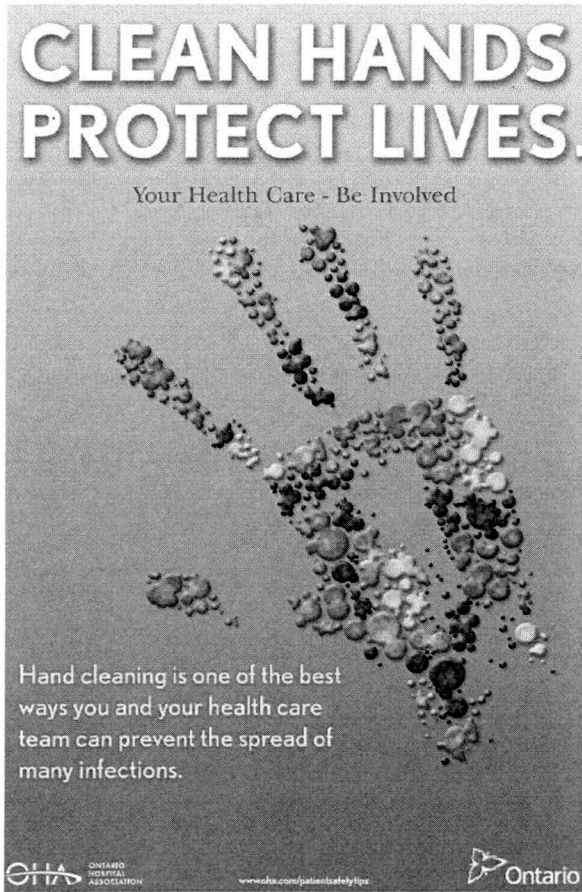

CLEAN HANDS PROTECT LIVES.

Your Health Care - Be Involved

Hand cleaning is one of the best ways you and your health care team can prevent the spread of many infections.

This poster and other tools and materials are available online for download.

Source: Ontario Hospital Association: *Just Clean Your Hands.* http://www.justcleanyourhands.ca/ (accessed May 20, 2009).

in Figures 5-1, (above) 5-2, and 5-3 (page 86), and many others are available online. For instance, information and tools for providers and patients are also available at the Institute for Healthcare Improvement Web site, http://www.ihi.org.

Infection-related Sentinel Events

Joint Commission requirements for ambulatory care recommend focusing attention on the prevention of the spread of health care–associated infection.

HAIs are major contributors to sentinel events. Historically, these infectious complications were considered inevitable consequences of health care interventions, but many HAIs are preventable. Key components to identify an HAI in an AHC setting include collecting data on infection rates, developing formal policies and procedures

Table 5-1. Tips from the CDC's Clean Hands Save Lives Campaign

Recommendations for Hand Hygiene

- When not visibly soiled, hands should be washed with an alcohol-based hand rub, or wash hands for a minimum of 15 seconds with warm water and antimicrobial or nonantimicrobial soap, taking care to rub all surfaces of the hands vigorously. Rinse and dry.

- When visibly soiled or contaminated with blood or other protein-based substance, body fluids, or spores, hands should be washed for a minimum of 15 seconds with warm water and antimicrobial or nonantimicrobial soap; take care to vigorously rub all surfaces of the hands. Rinse and dry.

- Wash hands or use an alcohol-based hand rub before putting on gloves and after removal of gloves; before and after direct contact with patients or medical equipment; if moving from a contaminated site to a noncontaminated site on the same patient; before and after eating or using the restroom; and after touching side rails, intravenous pumps or poles, bedside tables, linens, etc.

- Do not wear artificial nails or natural nails longer than 1/4 inch. Nail polish should have no chips.

- Use facility-approved hand lotions or creams to minimize irritation from frequent hand washing and/or decontamination.

Hand Washing with Soap and Water

- Advance paper towel from the dispenser before turning on the water to avoid touching the paper towel dispenser with clean, wet hands.

- Use facility-provided soap and warm (not hot) water and run the entire surface of both hands vigorously for at least 15 seconds.

- Rinse and leave the water running while drying hands with previously advanced paper towel.

- Turn the faucet off and open the bathroom door with a disposable paper towel.

Decontamination of Hands with Alcohol-Based Hand Rub

- Apply manufacturer recommended amount of alcohol-based product to the palm of one hand.

- Rub hands together vigorously, wetting all surfaces of both hands. Continue rubbing until hands are completely dry.

Source: Sandlin D: Did you wash your hands? Campaign. *J Perianesth Nur* 22:139–141, Apr. 2007.

Figure 5-2. How to Hand Wash Poster

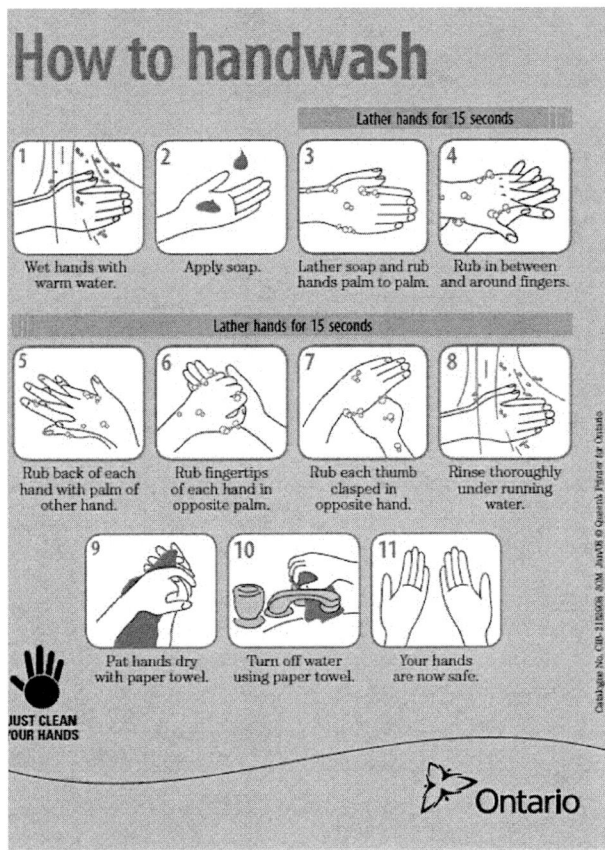

While lathering hands, sing "Happy Birthday" twice for the proper amount of time.

Source: Ontario Hospital Association: *Just Clean Your Hands.* http://www.justcleanyourhands.ca/ (accessed May 20, 2009).

Figure 5-3. How to Hand Rub Poster

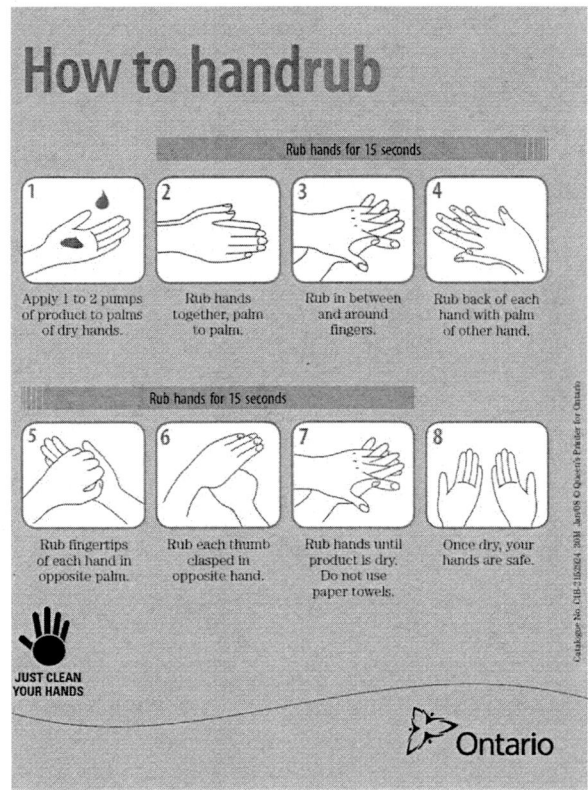

Rubbing and washing are different. Careful hygiene protects patients.

Source: Ontario Hospital Association: *Just Clean Your Hands.* http://www.justcleanyourhands.ca/ (accessed May 20, 2009).

to address the problem, and directing interventions to prevent infections.

AHC can improve infection prevention practices and control infection by taking the following steps[1]:

- Institute and enforce respiratory hygiene policies.
- Institute and enforce hand hygiene policies (as described above in this chapter).
- Immunize all staff.
- Establish policies that separate potentially contagious patients from the rest.
- Follow best practices to prevent SSIs (*see* the section on the SCIP program in this chapter beginning on page 88).

In the event of an HAI, an organization should evaluate the management of the patient in question by determining whether or not the patient's death or injury was unanticipated, and by conducting a root cause analysis (RCA). This multiuse health care tool is described below. The RCA should focus on managing the patient both before and after identifying the infection. If it is determined that the patient has an HAI, an IC professional (either on site or consulted) should participate in conducting a thorough and credible RCA to define, study, and identify the problem.

The investigation team should also include a leader with decision-making authority, a representative of frontline staff most involved in the care process, and individuals with diverse systems and process knowledge. The IC professional should determine any contributing process factors and then design and implement a plan for interim changes and, ultimately, a final revision of processes or policy. The tool on page 88 presents the steps for conducting an RCA. These guidelines can help staff when investigating a sentinel event or near-miss event.

Table 5-2. Best Practices for Conducting a Root Cause Analysis and Implementing an Action Plan

Conducting the RCA

- Look for the actions and conditions that sourced the error or problem.
- Include the director of the area or division and any involved staff as participants in the RCA process. Involve trained and competent (that is, trained in RCA) staff. Do not invite managers, supervisors, or administrators unless they were directly involved in the process being studied.
- Involve a strong leader who will facilitate and keep the discussion on track.
- Use a blame-free approach to assure participants there will be no reprisal. Address any individual performance problems (as opposed to systems-related problems) outside the RCA forum.
- Make the discussion timely, and do not jump to conclusions when first starting the process; analysis should be postponed until all information is collected.
- RCA is a tool of questions. Ask these questions:
    —What exactly was the adverse event?
    —What was the chain of events that resulted in the adverse event?
    —Was this event preventable?
    —What were the errors that led to the adverse event?
    —What were the root causes, both direct and indirect, that led to the errors and the adverse event?
    —Did any of the errors involved relate to core systems failures?
    —Do we need to redesign these systems?
    —What are the lessons learned?
- Because staff may not be able to describe the exact process leading to an error, wait to hold that discussion until those who were present for the error (if that is the case) are present at the discussion table.
- Conduct an analysis, backed up by findings in the scientific literature.
- Establish a way to communicate progress to senior leadership.
- Offer education to staff, including nonclinical staff.
- Create a high-level work plan that includes target dates, responsibilities, and measurement strategies.
- Sort and analyze the cause list.
- For each cause, determine which process(es) and system(s) it is part of and the interrelationship of its causes.
- Determine whether the causes are special causes, common causes, or both.
- Begin designing and implementing changes while finishing the RCA.
- After the analysis is finished, create an action plan.

Implementing the action plan

- Share best-practice findings with the entire organization. For example, changes in a particular surgical suite should also be implemented in other areas where procedures are performed.
- Send copies of the RCA action plan, which should not mention individual names, to each person responsible for an action.
- Send a copy of the action plan to administration and the quality review committee, if there is one, immediately after the final action is implemented.
- Conduct a trial of the action plan to see where any issues may break down. Don't "close the loop" on selected corrective actions; continue to monitor the processes.
- Establish a way to communicate progress to senior leadership.
- Offer education to staff, including nonclinical staff.
- Progress to create a high-level work plan that includes target dates, responsibilities, and measurement strategies.
- Assess progress periodically.
- Repeat activities (for example, brainstorming) as needed.
- Be thorough and credible.
- Focus improvements on the larger system(s).
- Redesign processes to eliminate the root cause(s).
- Measure and assess the new design.

Sources: Modified from Joint Commission Resources: Conducting root cause analyses of infection-related sentinel events. *The Joint Commission Perspectives on Patient Safety* 8:1–5, Jul. 2008. Do your root cause analyses fail to improve safety? Take these steps. *Hosp Peer Rev* 33:73–76, Jun. 2008.

TOOL: Root Cause Analysis

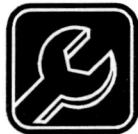

Root Cause Analysis (RCA) can be a valuable and effective tool in the quality and safety toolbox, useful in many areas of health care.[9] Employing RCA can be crucial to keep near misses from developing into adverse events, and adverse events from growing into sentinel events. Proper use of RCA can help move staff beyond the immediate cause of a deviation or error to an understanding of the root causes.

Examples of circumstances in which RCA methods can be used include following a surgical fire (see Chapter 4, "Surgical Safety"); IC, as described above; or with problems pertaining to radiation and magnetic resonance imaging (see Chapter 6, "Environment and Equipment").

The RCA methodology is sensitive and specific, allowing users to identify process details of failure modes. This facilitates targeting action plans that will most guarantee eradicating the roots of errors. Table 5-2, page 87, presents best practices for employing RCA and implementing an action plan. A tool for conducting an RCA is available on the Joint Commission Web site.

Tracking the Data

Typically ASCs and office-based surgery (OBS) practices experience low postsurgical infection rates. As reported by the Ambulatory Surgery Center Association (ASCA), data indicated a 0% rate of postsurgical wound infection in 76% of the 600 freestanding centers reporting in 2007.[1] However, the growth of surgeries performed in freestanding surgery centers or office-based practices over the past two decades has led to a call for greater surveillance.

An ambulatory organization's IC leaders or committee should establish and implement an IC program to enable staff members to do the following:
- Regularly monitor all procedures performed for compliance with safe IC practices
- Adjust spacing of clinical equipment to decrease the risk of contamination during the performance of surgical procedures
- Monitor infection rates following all surgical procedures in any location in the organization
- Provide a summary of all surgical procedures performed

- Compile a list of infections resulting after surgical procedures in the surgical and patient-care areas by type of procedure and surgeon
- Track all infections following surgical procedures to develop a comprehensive infection monitoring policy as a measurable outcome
- Provide organizational leaders and managers with a summary of incident reports to track any trends in infectious complications of surgical procedures that may not be identified through the usual monitoring mechanisms (for example, incident reporting)

The SCIP program to reduce surgical complications, and other means of monitoring outcomes, are discussed below.

SCIP Program for Surgical Site Infection

In 2003, in an effort to improve surgical care in hospitals nationwide, a national partnership of public and private health care organizations launched a project to reduce surgical complications to 25% by the year 2010.[10] The Surgical Care Improvement Project (SCIP) was initiated by the CMS and the CDC. The project, which is for hospitals only, does contain principles that are applicable to AHC. The project is coordinated through a steering committee of 10 leading organizations. More than 20 additional organizations provided technical expertise and resources to ensure that the SCIP measures were fully supported by evidence-based research.

Partnering to prevent surgical complications involves surgeons, anesthesiologists, perioperative nurses and other clinical staff, pharmacists, IC personnel, and executives and administrators. Although some surgical complications are unavoidable, care can be improved by adhering to evidence-based practice recommendations and designing systems of care with redundant safeguards. For example, delivering antibiotics to a patient within one hour of beginning surgery can dramatically cut SSI rates. Yet this practice is far from universally applied.

SCIP gives providers effective strategies to reduce a number of surgical complications. One of the top complications is SSIs. The good news is that 40% to 60% of SSIs can be prevented.

SCIP tracks four areas, one of which is health care–acquired infections, and includes seven Infection Prevention Process Measures. Of these, the following measures

Table 5-3. Outcomes Monitoring Project Percentage Tracking Quality Measures

Percentage of ASCs Formally Tracking and Documenting Clinical Indicators

Clinical Indicators	Yes	No
Unexpected complications	95.5%	3.5%
Postsurgical wound infection	97.4%	2.6%
Unscheduled direct transfers	95.0%	2.0%
Patient death	95.5%	4.5%
Return to surgery	94.4%	5.6%
Wrong site, side, procedure, implant, patient	95.4%	4.6%
Prophylactic IV antibiotic administration on time	51.0%	49.0%
Hair removal by clippers or depilatory cream	21.7%	76.3%

In 2008 the participants in the ASCA project monitored these eight measures.

Source: Ambulatory Surgery Center Association (ASCA). Outcomes Monitoring Project Center, 2008.

are germane to ambulatory care:

- SCIP INF 1: Prophylactic antibiotic received within one hour prior to surgical incision
- SCIP INF 2: Prophylactic antibiotic selection for surgical patients
- SCIP INF 3: Prophylactic antibiotics discontinued within 24 hours after surgery end time (48 hours for cardiac patients)
- SCIP INF 6: Surgery patients with appropriate hair removal

The U.S. Department of Health & Human Services recently announced plans to launch a new IC survey tool for ASCs.[11] The tool, developed in consultation with the CDC, incorporates a case tracer methodology that tracks the patient's care from admission to discharge. Updated outcomes information specific to ASCs is posted at http://www.ascquality.org/qualityreport.html. This information will be supplemented with additional data from the ASCA outcomes monitoring project. This tool will be applied to all Medicare-certified ASCs, including those using the deemed status option through The Joint Commission.

Outcomes Monitoring

Patient safety strategies generally focus on medical injury and medical errors. By reviewing patient outcomes, leaders and staff can measure medical injury and medical errors. Because outcomes can be used to identify and focus on a problem after harm or injury has occurred, ambulatory organizations and settings can use outcomes monitoring to effect better procedure policies.[12]

Use a performance improvement team process to involve all individuals in contact with the patient during an ambulatory surgical procedure. Adopt a methodology to focus on injury prevention and study the problem, reviewing all steps involved in ambulatory procedures. Develop a comprehensive procedure sum-

mary for all levels of care at the organization. Then involve all stakeholders in the process to achieve buy-in and to ensure greater success.

The Outcomes Monitoring Project launched by the ASCA provides benchmarks for 38 key indicators, allowing participating ASCs to compare their specific data with national performance statistics on 34 indicators, including clinical outcomes.[13] Participants represent 46 U.S. states, and 60% of them work in multi-specialty practices. They also represent a wide variation in terms of specialty, payer, years in operation, and ASC size. Participation is free for ASCA members, with an annual deadline for application. Participants receive data in quarterly reports. For 2007, the chart presented in Table 5-3, above, shows the percentage of outcome measures the ASCs are tracking.

Benchmarking for OBS is more difficult. Although no specific project has yet been launched to track outcomes in OBS settings, individual specialty societies and organizations may maintain their own benchmarking systems. According to one benchmarking study compiled by Validare, Inc., surgical infections appear to be on the rise at OBS practices. Specifically, in 2006, the number of OBS organizations recording no infections decreased from 49% to 40%, while the number of those reporting more than four infections rose from 20% to 25%.[14] On a positive note, a smaller percentage of clinical staff is routinely administering preprocedural/surgical antibiotics. In 2006, 35% of respondents routinely administered such antibiotics, compared with 45% in 2005.[14] Other issues that the study revealed include the increased use of alcohol-based rubs, but in combination with soap products, and the use of appropriate decontaminant and sterilization techniques.

Difficulties arise because OBS licensing and requirements differ from state to state. Thus far, causes of safety problems in OBS are shown to be multifactorial. Undergoing an accreditation process, such as that of The Joint Commission, encourages safeguards to be taken, but more data are needed to provide evidence for statistically significant results.[15,16]

Tracking data and outcomes monitoring are useful in many areas of AHC besides IC.

References

1. Joint Commission Resources: Preventing infection in ambulatory and office-based surgery centers. *Joint Comm Perspect Patient Safety* 9:1–11, May 2009.

2. Nihill D.: *Infection Control in a Changing Environment.* Association of Professionals in Infection Control and Epidemiology (APIC). PowerPoint presentation. "Infection Control and Epidemiology II: Clinical Problem Solving in Multiple Practice Settings" course, Dallas TX, Mar. 2005.

3. Thompson N.D., et al.: Nonhospital health care–associated hepatitis B and C virus transmission: United States, 1998–2008. *Ann Intern Med* 150:33–39, Jan. 6, 2009.

4. Surgistrategies: *Nev. Health District Finds 77 More Hep. C Cases.* May 9, 2008. http://www.surgistrategies.com/hotnews/more-nevada-hepatitis-c.html (accessed May 20, 2009).

5. Kuehn B.M.: Poor infection control fuels hepatitis in nonhospital health care facilities. *JAMA* 301:589, Feb. 11, 2009.

6. Association for Professionals in Infection Control and Epidemiology (APIC): Reduce your Risk of Infection Before an Ambulatory Procedure. 2009. http://www.apic.org/Content/NavigationMenu3/InformationCenter/OutpatientCare/Reduce_your_risk_of_infection_before_an_ambulatory_procedure.pdf (accessed May 20, 2009).

7. Centers for Disease Control and Prevention: Guideline for Hand Hygiene in Health-Care Settings: Recommendations of the Healthcare Infection Control Practices Advisory Committee and the HICPAC/SHEA/APIC/ IDSA Hand Hygiene Task Force. *MMWR* 51:1-56, Oct. 25, 2002.

8. Centers for Disease Control and Prevention, Department of Health and Human Services: *Epidemiology and Prevention of Vaccine-Preventable Diseases,* 10th ed. Skills Checklist for Immunization. Appendix D, page D-14, 2008. http://www.cdc.gov/vaccines/Pubs/pinkbook/downloads/appendices/appdx-full-d.pdf (accessed May 13, 2009).

9. Do your root causes analyses fail to improve safety? Take these steps. *Hosp Peer Rev* 33:73–76, Jun. 2008.

10. Centers for Disease Control and Prevention: SCIP—Surgical Care Improvement Project. www.cdc.gov/ (accessed Mar. 7, 2009).

11. HHS announces infection control surveys for ASCs. *Surgistrategies.* Apr. 2, 2009. http://www.surgistrategies.com/hotnews/hhs-asc-infect-control-surveys.html (accessed May 19, 2009).

12. Kleinpeter M.A.: Standardizing ambulatory care procedures in a public hospital system to improve patient safety. In Henriksen K., et al. (ed.): *Advances in Patient Safety: From Research to Implementation.* Vol. 4: Programs, Tools, and Products. Rockville, MD: Agency for Healthcare Research and Quality and the Department of Defense-Health Affairs. National Library of Medicine. http://www.ncbi.nlm.nih.gov/books/bv.fcgi?rid=aps.section.6867#6887 (accessed Mar. 2, 2009).

13. Ambulatory Surgery Center Association: Outcomes Monitoring Project Center. *FASA Update* Sep.–Oct. 2007. http://www.ascassociation.org/outcomes/ (accessed Mar. 3, 2009).

14. Joint Commission Resources: Case study: Reducing surgical infections at office-based surgery organizations. *Jt Comm Benchmark* 10:10–11, Jan.–Feb. 2008.

15. Coldiron B.M., Healy C., Bene N.I.: Office surgery incidents: What seven years of Florida data show us. *Dermatol Surg* 34:285–292, Mar. 2008.

16. Vila H., et al.: Comparative outcomes analysis of procedures performed in physician offices and ambulatory surgery centers. *Arch Surg* 138:991–995, Sep. 2003.

Chapter 6

ENVIRONMENT AND EQUIPMENT

Regardless of whether an ambulatory health care (AHC) facility is classified as a "health care occupancy" or a "business occupancy" (*see* the box below), the environment where care is provided and the equipment used to provide that care must be safe. The Joint Commission requirements are based on the occupancy classification; that is, the intended use of the building or portion occupied by the organization as per the *Life Safety Code®*.* Any plan that the organization outlines for managing the ambulatory environment of care (EC) is vital and should be integrated into an organization's overall care processes.

The six major considerations in the EC, as outlined in Joint Commission standards are as follows:
1. Safety and security
2. Hazardous materials and waste management
3. Emergency preparedness
4. Life safety
5. Management of medical equipment
6. Utilities management

Plans and policies do not need to be complex or burdensome, but rather, their scope, performance, and effectiveness can be simple, flexible, and relevant to the particular organization's patients, staff, and visitors.[1]

The ambulatory care setting's environmental design presents challenges for establishing and maintaining safety. Leaders at the site should conduct regular safety walks to observe potential safety risks and to make it known to staff that they wholeheartedly promote a culture of safety. Besides emphasizing the importance of safety to staff, these walks (or rounds) produce data regarding safety hazards for which actions should be designed and taken. Examples include the following[1,2]:

- A scale left in a walkway or hallway that might precipitate falls
- Equipment blocks or barriers causing workflow workarounds
- Safety risks in exam rooms, such as sharps containers within children's reach
- Hand hygiene materials and equipment (gel dispensers, sinks) that are not easily accessible
- Equipment that is not sterilized but may carry pathogens; for example, armrests, uncovered portions of headrests

To best manage your EC, do the following[3]:
- Collect information about deficiencies and opportunities for improvement in environment.
- Analyze identified environmental issues.
- Develop recommendations for resolving them.

What is the difference between "ambulatory health care occupancy" and "business health care occupancy"?

Ambulatory Health Care Facilities: A building or part of a building used to provide services or treatment to four or more patients at the same time that meets the criteria of either (a) or (b) below.

(a) Facilities that provide, on an outpatient basis, treatment for patients incapable of taking action for self-preservation under emergency conditions without assistance from others.

(b) Facilities that provide, on an outpatient basis, surgical treatment requiring general anesthesia.

Example: A surgi-center with three operating rooms and six recovery beds that normally has four or more patients under anesthesia or recovering.

All other settings for outpatients are business health care occupancy. Example: A primary care clinic where only local anesthetics are used.

---

* *Life Safety Code®* is a registered trademark of the National Fire Protection Association, Inc., Quincy, MA.

■ Implement recommendations to improve the environment.

■ Monitor how effectively the recommendations are implemented.

In an ambulatory surgical center (ASC), best managing the EC would include ensuring that there is a dependable electrical and ventilation system and that it has sufficient capacity to pipe in gases appropriate to anesthesia use[1] (*see* "Emergency Power Sources" in Chapter 4, beginning on page 65).

It is recommended that a staff member be designated to be accountable for follow-up on any identified patient safety environmental risks for repairs, replacements, solutions, and adjustments. In a larger ambulatory care organization, a safety officer should be designated and should lead a committee responsible for the EC.[1] The issues addressed by the safety officer/committee should take into account the organization's varied work shifts and hours of operation. The designated individual or group is expected to develop, implement, and maintain a comprehensive organizationwide safety program. The intent of the process is to ensure that a quality EC is provided and that staff are alerted to issues and processes that result in a safe and effective care environment.

Each organization should know the structural features of its own buildings and spaces. Some ambulatory settings go through cycles of remodeling and expanding their existing facilities. During these periods of renovation and innovation, staff can observe and plan for patient (and staff) movement, patient visibility, infection prevention and control (IC), and standardization. Throughout any design or redesign processes, the entire health care team—from clinical to clerical—should be asked to contribute because their experience in the work-place can greatly affect improvements across the board.

Environmental and equipment-related safety concerns that are of particular relevance in AHC include emergency management plans, steam sterilization, imaging safety, radiation safety, and workflow redesign. Each are discussed in the following sections.

TOOL: Patient Safety Environmental Rounds

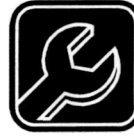

Patient safety environmental rounds are one of the best ways to gather information and data on how safety is being maintained in your facility or institution. The University of Michigan Hospitals and Health System in Ann Arbor, Michigan, use environmental rounds to help establish a culture of safety across the organization. The health system includes a number of ambulatory clinics and health centers, such as a Cardiovascular Center and a Cancer Center, and three ambulatory surgery sites. During these rounds, management and frontline staff work together to identify hazards and take actions to reduce or eliminate them.[4]

The Private Diagnostic Clinics (PDC) of Duke University Medical Center, Durham, North Carolina, is composed of 52 freestanding, non–hospital-based ambulatory care clinics that provide specialty and primary care in locations across North Carolina and one in Virginia. Since 2001, the PDC have been conducting mock tracers. However, in 2003 the PDC began The Patient Safety Rounds (PSR) project, to improve quality and safety.[5]

For example, a clinic physician and a clinic staff leader will follow the exact route that the patient must take through the medical experience, looking for barriers and safety issues both outside and inside. The project team uses a formal checklist to mark areas needing improvement. For example, one clinic noticed a problem with its electronic doors, which were closing too early, sometimes striking patients. After opportunities for improvement are identified and reported, the clinic manager then has two weeks in which to submit an action plan to leadership. The team meets monthly with managers from various clinics to share with them the results of the current patient safety rounds.

Emergency Management Plans

The organization should develop policies and procedures for emergency management. These plans must be designed to ensure that patients can receive high-quality care in a safe environment, despite any called emergencies (*see also* Chapter 4, "Surgical Safety").

A plan should address handling hazardous materials, waste spills and exposures, and other emergencies.[1] These incidents may be generic (cleaning a spill of blood or body fluid) or specific (handling a mercury spill or radiation exposure). All plans should be flexible and dynamic.

The Joint Commission standards for emergency preparedness address the ambulatory care organization's need to develop a clear, concise, practical, and preestablished organizationwide plan. This plan should be simple enough to be implemented alone or in conjunction with communitywide disaster efforts. For example, emergency preparedness must include a plan for hazardous materials incidents in the community.[1]

Emergency preparedness focuses on a readiness plan for three main areas: facility preparedness, staff preparedness, and patient management, as described below.

Facility preparedness focuses on the building elements (structural and nonstructural) that must be operable for staff to effectively perform patient care. This includes space requirements, supplies, utilities, communication systems, and security.

Staff preparedness involves staff requirements (any additional staff in an emergency event), establishing staff responsibilities, designating staff roles (based on experience and availability), and education and orientation programs for staff, including key communication requirements in critical stress periods.[1]

Well-coordinated patient management is paramount in the event of disaster. During a disaster event, patients already at the facility must be able to continue to receive required care. This will include modifying schedules for surgical and other procedures, and a plan to determine which services, if any, must be discontinued. Special procedures must be developed to determine how patients will be moved or evacuated from the facility. A comprehensive plan also addresses discharge planning, relocation, and medical record keeping and tagging.

Steam Sterilization

The Association for the Advancement of Medical Instrumentation (AAMI) defines *rapid-cycle steriliza-tion*, a term that more accurately describes the process that's commonly referred to as flash sterilization, as the steam sterilization of patient care items for immediate use.[6]

The requirements for the steam sterilization process are evolving. The 2009 Healthcare Infection Control Practices Advisory Committee (HICPAC) guidelines, published in November 2008, outline more detail for ambulatory organizational requirements. (The HICPAC guidelines are available on the CDC Web site at http://www.cdc.gov/ncidod/dhqp/pdf/guidelines/Disinfection_Nov_2008.pdf.)

Consider the following parameters for determining when steam sterilization should be used[6]:
- When proper work practices for cleaning, decontaminating, inspecting, and arranging instruments in the sterilizing tray or containers are carefully followed
- When the physical configuration of the department or area facilitates direct delivery of sterilized items
- When staff follow and audit standard procedures for personnel safety and aseptic handling of sterilized instruments during transfer of use

Steam sterilization is associated with several potential shortcomings that may affect safety and quality. These are presented in Table 6-1, page 94.

TASS and Steam Sterilization

A particular concern for using rapid-cycle sterilization is the development of toxic anterior segment syndrome (TASS), a rare, potentially devastating complication of routine intraocular surgery.[7] TASS occurs when a noninfectious toxic agent enters the anterior segment of the eye, causing an inflammatory reaction. Severe cases of TASS lead to permanent injury; that is, if TASS symptoms are still present six weeks after surgery, the eye is not likely to recover. Although early diagnosis and treatment can prevent permanent damage, TASS is often mistakenly diagnosed as infectious endophthalmitis, for which treatment is completely different.

Methods to prevent TASS are listed in Table 6-2, page 94. (TASS guidelines from the American Society of Cataract and Refractive Surgery can be found online at http://www.ascrs.org/TASS.)

Table 6-1. Potential Risks of the Rapid-Cycle Process

- Instruments are not cleaned before sterilization and use. This presents an increased risk of recontamination and health care–acquired infection (HAI).

- Rapid-cycle sterilization is performed near or in the operating room by staff whose primary focus is patient care—not instrument sterilization.

- Documentation and records associated with rapid-cycle sterilized instruments—unlike instruments processed using traditional steam sterilization cycles—are typically incomplete, if not entirely absent, which precludes adequately tracking "flashed" instruments.

- Some manufacturers of surgical instruments (and implants) contraindicate steam sterilization. The rapid heating and cooling of its rapid, high-temperature cycle can cause chipping, flaking, and other types of damage to some types of surgical instruments.

- Steam sterilization has been a concern regarding whether the process damages ophthalmic instruments, allowing pieces of the instrument's surface to be introduced into the eye during cataract surgery, increasing the risk for toxic anterior segment syndrome (TASS).

TIP

- Don't wash instruments in your facility's dishwasher. Particularly in a physician's office, staff members may use a dishwasher to sterilize medical equipment. This process does not meet the Centers for Disease Control and Prevention's sterilization guidelines for high-level disinfection.

Guidelines for Steam Sterilization

As recommended by the AAMI and the Association of periOperative Registered Nurses (AORN), a number of steps should be taken to follow guidelines for using steam sterilization. Tips for using rapid-cycle sterilization are presented in Table 6-3, page 95. This list will help staff recognize when and how to properly use rapid-cycle sterilization.

The Joint Commission has been in discussion with multiple professional and trade organizations regarding the common and proper use of sterilization using steam in ambulatory care and office-based surgery (OBS) set-

Table 6-2. General Principles of Cleaning and Sterilizing Intraocular Surgical Instruments

- Develop written procedures for instrument cleaning and sterilization for your facility.

- Train your staff in your cleaning and sterilization techniques, validate competency, and conduct periodic reviews.

- Allow adequate time to complete all the steps involved in cleaning and sterilizing your instruments.

- Keep your surgical instruments moist until the cleaning process begins.

- Remove all debris.

- Use the quality and volume of water for suspending detergents and cleaning and rinsing instruments in the ways your manufacturers specify.

- Follow your detergent and instrument manufacturers' directions for using the products they supply.

- During rinsing, remove all cleaning agents and all debris loosened during the cleaning process.

Source: *FASA Update.* TASS prevention at your ASC. May–Jun. 2007.

tings. Recently, some decisions have been made that will have an impact on the interpretation of standards and the survey process. The Joint Commission released a statement on steam sterilization in June 2009,[8] from which this discussion is derived. In reviewing this method of sterilization, several issues have emerged, including nomenclature, indications, and process issues.

Flash sterilization is the most common term used to describe certain types of steam sterilization that do not utilize a full cycle (also known as a terminal cycle). Originally, flash sterilization meant sterilizing unwrapped instruments using steam for 3 minutes, at 270°F at 27 to 28 pounds of pressure. Over the past several decades, a number of improvements have been made to this process, such as longer exposure of the instruments to steam, the use of special trays and packs to hold and protect the instruments, and the routine use of biological indicators. To help sort out confusion about nomenclature, this discussion refers only to steam sterilization as defined (3 minutes at 270°F at 27 to 28 pounds of pressure).

Indication-related issues involve selecting the sterilization cycle or method. Examples of potential safety

<table>
<tr><td>

Table 6-3. Tips to Help Avoid Complications Associated with Rapid-Cycle Sterilization

1. Enforce protocols.
Define the rules for steam sterilization at your facility and establish appropriate protocols for everyone to follow. Require use of a steam sterilization log.

2. Build more efficient instrument sets.
Inventory your facility's instruments and determine those that are most frequently used. Streamlined instrument sets should be built to include only those instruments. Fewer instruments per set allows for faster overall processing. With streamlined sets, money isn't wasted on rarely used instruments.

3. Dedicate someone to instrument reprocessing.
Ensure that all instruments are sterilized through proper reprocessing by dedicating someone to this responsibility. Patient safety is an important measure for all facilities, and reprocessing instruments is a crucial element of a sterile and safe environment. This individual should monitor the process your organization uses, including training.

4. Seek outside support.
If your budget or systems can't keep up with your demands, seek outside help. Certain companies can serve as outsourced sterilization services or even provide sterile instruments on a just-in-time and charge-by-use basis.

5. If you are going to use rapid-cycle sterilization, do it right.
You may want to use closed sterilization containers or a patented system so instruments are protected from contamination from autoclave to point of use. Such a system is easy to use, sterilization is fully validated, and instruments can be transported through nonsterile areas safely and within guidelines.

Source: Excerpted from Schaag J.: Quick guide to flash sterilization considerations. *ICT: Infection Control Today,* Apr. 16, 2008.

</td></tr>
</table>

issues would be a high percentage of steam sterilization using less than a full sterilization cycle or the exclusive use of this process for certain types of instruments.

Process-related issues involve the way a given sterilization method is executed. Examples of potential safety issues would be failure to adequately clean the instruments before sterilization (rinsing is rarely enough to properly remove soil from instruments; meticulous cleaning is needed), lack of chemical indicators, and

transporting uncovered instruments back to the operating room after they have been sterilized.

Based on discussions with experts in the field, professional organizations, and government organizations, The Joint Commission has decided to refocus its survey efforts on all the critical processes included in sterilization. If a complete and effective process of sterilization is used, it will be considered an effective sterilization method. Therefore, surveyors will review the critical steps of disinfection and sterilization to determine if the process is appropriate. The three critical steps of reprocessing are the following:

1. *Cleaning and decontamination.* All visible soil must be removed prior to sterilization because steam and other sterilants cannot penetrate soil, particularly organic matter. Manufacturers' instructions are available for all instruments; these include directions for the cleaning and decontamination process. Some smooth metal instruments may be easily brushed clean, while complex products may require disassembly and special cleaning techniques. Many manufacturers specify that an enzymatic soak be used as well.

2. *Sterilization.* Most sterilization is accomplished via steam, but other methods are also available. Steam sterilization of all types, including flashing, must meet parameters (time, temperature, and pressure) specified by both the manufacturer of the sterilizer, the maker of any wrapping or packaging, and the manufacturer of the surgical instrument. In addition to these instructions, parametric, chemical, and biological controls must be used as designed and directed by their manufacturers.

3. *Storage or return to the sterile field.* Each newly sterilized instrument must be carefully protected to ensure that it is not recontaminated. For full steam sterilization cycles, packs of instruments are wrapped and sealed. Instruments subjected to steam sterilization using methods other than full-cycle sterilization may be transported in "flash pans" or other devices specifically designed for preventing contamination during and after the steam process.

For more information, see the *2008 Guideline for Disinfection and Sterilization in Healthcare Facilities* from the HICPAC of the Centers for Disease Control and Prevention online at http://www.cdc.gov/ncidod/dhqp/pdf/guidelines/Disinfection_Nov_2008.pdf.

Figure 6-1. Example Steam Sterilization Documentation Log

STERILIZER #_____ FLASH STERILIZATION LOG DEPARTMENT_____

Date	Description of items	Doctor	Room #	Item	Exposure time	Result of CI	BI run? (Y/N)	Reason item(s) flashed	Patient ID #	Items removed by

Keeping a steam sterilization log provides a means of carefully observing practices.

Source: Chobin N. Are you up to speed on flash sterilization? *OR Manager* 23:17–18, Mar. 2007.

If you do use rapid-cycle sterilization, adhere to the following strategies[7]:
- Monitor what is being steamed and why.
- Ensure proper cleaning.
- Ensure direct delivery to point of use with the physical layout.
- Monitor practices for aseptic handling and personnel safety during transport of sterilized items.
- Avoid burns in patients (ensure ample cooling time before use of a flashed item).

Best practice for proper documentation of medical instrument reprocessing includes the following[7]:
- The sterilizer identification and cycle number
- The item(s) that was sterilized
- The temperature of the cycle
- The type of cycle used (prevacuum or gravity)
- The identification of the staff member processing the item(s)
- The date and time of the cycle
- The results of the chemical integrator
- Any process indicator used
- The patient identification number and patient name for traceability purposes

An example of a steam sterilization documentation log tool that could be used is shown in Figure 6-1, above.

MRI Safety

Magnetic resonance imaging (MRI) has been a vital part of health care diagnostics since the 1970s. More than 10 million MRI scans are performed in the United States each year.[9] Using MRI has its risks, as outlined in a 2008 *Sentinel Event Alert* issued by The Joint Commission.[9]

In general, the following types of injury can and have occurred during the MRI scanning process[9]:

- Injury or complication related to equipment or device malfunction or failure caused by the magnetic field. For example, battery-powered devices (microinfusion pumps, monitors, and so on) may suddenly fail to operate, some programmable infusion pumps may perform erratically, and pacemakers and implantable defibrillators may not behave as programmed.
- Injury or complication due to failure to attend to patient support systems during the MRI. This is particularly true for patient sedation or anesthesia in MRI arenas. For example, if oxygen canisters or infusion pumps run out, airways or tubing can become dislodged, and staff must either leave the MRI area to retrieve a replacement or move the patient to an area where a replacement can be found.
- Acoustic injury from the loud knocking noise that the MRI scanner makes
- Adverse events related to administering MRI contrast agents
- Adverse events related to cryogen handling, storage, or inadvertent release in superconducting MRI system sites

Risk reduction strategies for the many ferromagnetic objects associated with MRI scanning are presented in Table 6-4 on this page. The list can help you prevent missile-effect accidents with scanners.

Safety-risk identifiers will include prediagnostic and preinterventional history taking, regular calibration checks of MRI equipment, and patient complaints and missed appointments.[9] Set priorities for managing risk exposure (*see* "Preventing Patient Overexposure," page 99). For example, if an MRI machine is malfunctioning, take it offline to eliminate the risk of harm to patients and staff. Requiring demonstrated competencies of staff prior to using new MRI equipment signifies a firm approach to risk prevention.

Another preventive strategy is to consider orienting/training fire department personnel, who may be called to respond to a fire, about MRI safety.

The Joint Commission recommendations and strategies for reducing MRI accidents and injuries are summarized in Table 6-5, page 98. For a full discussion of and citations for this topic, refer to *Sentinel Event*

Table 6-4. Risk Reduction Strategies in the MRI Suite

- Appoint a safety officer who is responsible for implementing and enforcing safety procedures in the MRI suite.
- Implement systems to support safe MRI practice such as written protocols and checklists, and periodically review and assess compliance with your organization's MRI policies, procedures, and protocols.
- As part of these protocols, allow maintenance and housekeeping personnel to enter the MRI suite only after proper safety education.
- Allow *no patient in the suite* when maintenance and housekeeping personnel are working in there.
- In general, do not bring any device or equipment into the MRI environment unless it is proven to be MR Safe or MR Conditional. The safety of "MR Conditional" items must be verified with the specific scanner and MR environment in which they will be used.

Source: The Joint Commission: Preventing accidents and injuries in the MRI suite. *Sentinel Event Alert 38*, Feb. 14, 2008.

Alert Issue 38.[9] In addition, the American College of Radiology published white papers in 2002 and 2004 on the subject of MRI safety. These are available online at http://www.acr.org.

As described in Chapter 5, every organization must have a unique and specialized infection prevention plan that meets its specific needs. In addition, each organization must initiate a risk assessment strategy and methods for evaluating the success of that strategy. As part of that comprehensive IC program, direct your attention to the cleaning and disinfection of equipment and other items in the MRI suite. This can particularly serve as a safeguard against the possibility of asymptomatic persons with methicillin-resistant *Staphylococcus aureus* contaminating items and equipment in the suite.[10]

Radiation Safety

Radiation is a mainstay in many ambulatory settings, existing in lasers, x-rays, fluoroscopy equipment, and some radioactive materials, such as implants. Although radiologists are trained to be extremely careful when administering radiation, perioperative staff can be exposed to radiation in a variety of ways, and, therefore,

---

Table 6-5. The Joint Commission Recommendations and Strategies for Reducing MRI Accidents and Injuries

■ Restrict access to all MRI sites by implementing the four zone concept as defined in the ACR Guidance Document for Safe MR Practices: 2007. The four zone concept provides for progressive restrictions in access to the MRI scanner:
—Zone I: General public
—Zone II: Unscreened MRI patients
—Zone III: Screened MRI patients and personnel
—Zone IV: Screened MRI patients under constant direct supervision of trained MR personnel

■ Use trained personnel to screen all nonemergent patients twice, providing two separate opportunities for them to answer questions about any metal objects they may have on them, any implanted devices, drug delivery patches, or tattoos, and any electrically, magnetically, or mechanically activated devices they may have. If the patient is unconscious or unable to answer questions, query the patient's family member or surrogate decision maker. If this person is unsure, use other means to determine if the patient has implants or other devices that could be negatively affected by the MRI scan (for example, look for scars or deformities, scrutinize the patient's history, use plain-film radiography, use ferromagnetic detectors to assist in the screening process, and so forth).

■ Ensure that the MRI technologist has the patient's complete and accurate medical history to ensure that the patient can be safely scanned. All implants should be checked against product labeling or manufacturer's literature specific to that implant; or peer-reviewed published data regarding the device or implant in question. Technologists should be provided with ready access to this information.

■ Have a specially trained staff person who is knowledgeable about the MRI environment accompany any patients, visitors, and other staff who are not familiar with the MRI environment inside the MRI suite at all times.

■ Annually, provide all medical and ancillary staff who may be expected to accompany patients to the MRI suite with safety education about the MRI environment and provide all staff and patients and their families with appropriate materials (for example, guidelines, brochure, poster) that explain the potential for accidents and adverse events in the MRI environment.

■ Take precautions to prevent patient burns during scanning, including the following:
—Ensure that no items (such as leads) are formed into a loop because magnetic induction can occur and cause burns.
—If the patient's body touches the bore of the MRI scanner, use nonconductive foam padding to insulate the patient's skin and tissues.
—Place a cold compress or ice pack on EKG leads, surgical staples, and tattoos that will be exposed to radiofrequency irradiation during the MR imaging process.

■ Only use equipment (for example, fire extinguishers, oxygen tanks, physiologic monitors, and aneurysm clips) that has been tested and approved for use during MRI scans.

■ Proactively plan for managing critically ill patients who require physiologic monitoring and continuous infusion of life-sustaining drugs while in the MRI suite.

■ Provide all MRI patients with hearing protection (that is, ear plugs).

■ Never attempt to run a cardiopulmonary arrest code or resuscitation within the MRI magnet room itself.

Source: The Joint Commission: Preventing accidents and injuries in the MRI suite. *Sentinel Event Alert 38,* Feb. 14, 2008.

---

require a special setting-specific orientation to what is expected and required. Radiation equipment as well as all other equipment must be considered for disinfecting as part of a comprehensive IC program.

There are two types of radiation: ionizing and non-ionizing. Both types of radiation can be found in an operating room. Ionizing radiation is a low-frequency form that can be found in microwaves, radios, and lasers. Nonionizing radiation includes higher-frequency radiation, such as that found in gamma rays and x-rays.

Although patients are at risk any time they are exposed to radiation, staff are also at risk. Staff can be exposed to radiation through inhalation, absorption, or injection.[9] As an organization, policies should be established for reducing risks associated with working around radiation. Although radiation-related risks in health care cannot be eliminated or prevented, they can be reduced in terms of frequency or severity. Some general risk-reduction strategies are presented in Table 6-6, page 99. In addition, a number of organizations, including the Centers for Disease Control and Prevention, Occupational Safety and Health Administration, Association of periOperative Registered Nurses, and Association for the Advancement of Medical Instrumentation, have excellent sources of information and tools for protecting both patients and staff.

TOOL: Mock Survey

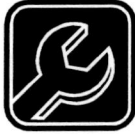

The mock survey helps staff maintain compliance between official surveys, but the most significant purpose of a mock survey is to check to see that the patient (and staff) is being protected and that, as it concerns patient safety, systems and structure are in place to enact behaviors that ultimately ensure that every element of the organization is safe. The most common tool in conducting a mock survey is to perform a patient or a system tracer to follow the care of a typical patient through the organization. Sidebar 6-1, pages 100–101, provides an example of a system tracer on the continuity of care and a narrative example of a patient tracer through an ASC.

Two areas for focus in reducing risks for patients are preventing overexposure to radiation and reducing the risk for computed tomography (CT)–induced medical device malfunction.

Preventing Patient Overexposure

Preventing patient overexposure to radiation dosing is an important safety consideration. Dose monitoring should include two checks by personnel. This is a particular concern when irradiating children. The "Image Gently"™ campaign is an effort to maintain safety in the area of pediatric imaging. In January 2008 the charter members of the Alliance for Radiation Safety in Pediatric Imaging (the Society for Pediatric Radiology, the American College of Radiology, the American Society of Radiologic Technologists, and the American Association of Physicists in Medicine) launched the Image Gently campaign. This is a national initiative to educate providers of pediatric imaging care about the importance of "child-sizing" radiation doses. Pediatric radiologists are urged to do the following[11]:

- "Child-size" the scan: This often reduces the amount of radiation used.
- Scan only when necessary.
- Scan only the indicated region.
- Scan once; multiphase scanning is usually not necessary in children.
- Be a team player.
- Involve medical physicists to monitor pediatric CT techniques.
- Involve technologists to optimize scanning.

Table 6-6. Risk Reduction Strategies for Working with Radiation

- Leave radioactive materials such as implants in their lead-shielded containers for as long as possible.
- Use gloves when handling radioactive materials.
- Wear protective masks and scrubs when working near radioactive materials that could be inhaled.
- Wear eye protection when working directly with highly radioactive materials.
- Use lead curtains when using high-frequency radiation such as x-rays. If for any reason you must place your hand behind the lead curtain, wear lead gloves.
- Keep a safe distance from any necessary shielding.
- Control access to areas where ionizing radiation is used.

Source: The Joint Commission: *Safety in the Operating Room.* Oakbrook Terrace, IL: Joint Commission Resources, 2006.

Computed Tomography Causing Medical Device Malfunction

Another aspect of radiation safety in ambulatory settings is the potential for CT scans to cause some implanted and external devices to malfunction. The list of devices includes cardiac pacemakers, implantable cardiac defibrillators, neurostimulators, drug infusion pumps (including insulin pumps), cochlear implants, and retinal implants.

Shocks or other stimuli can result from the device's direct exposure to high x-ray dose rates generated by some CT equipment. These malfunctions differ from those caused by MRI scanning, which result from strong electric and magnetic fields.

In its guidelines for CT scanning, the U.S. Food and Drug Administration recommends the following[12]:

- The operator uses CT scout views, an equipment setting that allows the operator to plot the locations where the subsequent slice images will be obtained. Scout views are also used to determine whether implanted or externally worn electronic medical devices are present.
- If a device is present, determine the location relative to the programmed scan range. If the device is in or immediately next to the programmed scan range, the operator should do the following:
  —Determine the type of device
  —If practical, try to move external devices out of

Sidebar 6-1. Sample Ambulatory Care Tracers

Continuity of Care System Tracer

A medical/dental provider undergoing a program-specific continuity of care tracer should ensure that the following is taking place:

- Develop a tracking system within the organization to make sure follow-up occurs in a timely manner for all adverse test results.
- Test the tracking system by randomly selecting patients and tracing the flow of communications from the time the physician or licensed independent practitioner orders the test to when action is taken based on the results.

The surveyor selects a patient who had one or more results for a laboratory or diagnostic test. The surveyor then follows how the process flows within the organization from the point at which the test was ordered, the performance of the test, to when the results are reported, to what, if any, action is taken. The surveyor will speak with staff such as nursing staff, the physician, the patient (if available), and laboratory staff.

A particular area that the surveyor should explore is how the care is coordinated and adequately communicated among care providers, particularly if the patient has to be referred to different specialties due to test results. Sample questions that could be asked in this scenario include the following:

- Can you describe your process for ordering a test and reporting the results? What is your organizational policy on time frames and staff involvement?
- I see that Mrs. Jones had an abnormal Pap smear result noted here in her record. Can you describe the normal process for handling such a result?
- Can you describe the communication process for ordering, performing, and reporting test results?

Patient Tracer in an Ambulatory Surgery Center

Surveyors conduct tracers during an on-site accreditation survey to assess how well an ambulatory care organization's systems and processes function to deliver safe, high-quality care, treatment, and services. By following a patient's experience or a system's function through a health care organization, surveyors are provided with an in-depth look at day-to-day operations and can ask staff relevant questions about how they deliver care. Although the surveyor is making the necessary links between actual care delivery and Joint Commission standards during tracer activity, staff members need only to understand and communicate clearly about their own work and how they carry it out.

In the following tracer narrative, a surveyor follows a patient through her surgical experience at an ASC. The narrative includes some example questions that could

be asked at specific points during the tracer. Please keep in mind that while the following narrative does represent a tracer that could take place in one type of ambulatory care setting, tracers are unique. No two tracers are alike. The following tracer is provided as an example only and may not represent all the tracers that may occur during an on-site survey.

Note: *The following tracer example is written from the perspective of a surveyor and as such is a first-person narrative.*

I conducted this tracer at a busy suburban ambulatory surgical center. I began the tracer with the selection of a particular patient who was receiving sinus surgery in the surgical center that day. Based on information in her clinical record, the patient I selected was elderly, undergoing her first sinus surgery, and was dealing with some health issues relating to Type 2 diabetes. At the time of selection, the patient had arrived in the surgical center and was being prepped for surgery. I began my tracer by visiting the registration desk of the surgical center and approached staff members to ask them about their registration process for this surgery patient. ["I see you registered Mrs. P for sinus surgery this morning. Could you explain the process that you followed with her?"]

After discussing the documentation that the patient was asked to complete—medical history and a list of medications used—I asked the registration staff member how staff ensure the patient's privacy while registering the patient. ["When you asked for insurance information or other protected health information that would be entered into the computer, how did you do that in a way that protected Mrs. P's privacy?"] The staff member explained the process and then showed me the Health Insurance Portability and Accountability Act (HIPAA) and other privacy-related documents. I then asked how they communicate and discuss any financial questions with the patient and family member. ["How did you discuss financial obligations and issues with the patient and her family member?"] While listening to the answer, I also observed another staff member register a different patient for surgery.

I walked into the preoperative preparation area and introduced myself to one of the nurses on staff. I explained that I was tracing Mrs. P's experience while she underwent surgery at the center that morning and asked to be introduced to the nurse who was assigned to Mrs. P's case. I then asked the preoperative nurse what his process was to assess and prepare Mrs. P for surgery. ["I see you were working with Mrs. P this

(continued on page 101)

Sidebar 6-1. Sample Ambulatory Tracers (continued)

morning. Could you tell me what steps you took to prepare and assess Mrs. P for surgery?"] I next asked the nurse what he did with the preadmission paperwork completed by the patient. ["What was your process for handling Mrs. P's preadmission paperwork?"] I then asked the nurse about his education and training experiences at the center and how his performance was assessed. The nurse replied that his last training was 18 months ago and covered some changes in procedure relating to assessment and history and physical. I later asked the administrator for a copy of this nurse's personnel file to review training, licensure, and other documentation. ["May I see the personnel file for this nurse? How and where do you document all training and competencies? How does your organization assess the competency of its staff?"]

When Mrs. P was in the postoperative area, I received permission to speak with her. I explained the purpose of my visit ["I am a surveyor from The Joint Commission and we assess organizations against a set of high-quality standards to ensure that they are delivering safe, high-quality care. I am here at the request of the organization for a periodic, unannounced assessment of their services."] I then asked the patient what her experiences had been with the organization. ["How did the center provide education to you for today's surgery? Were you informed about the risks and outcomes of the procedure? What did they tell you to expect after the procedure? Were you provided with information about the physician who would perform your surgery? Did the center share any information on privacy and safety issues? Have your questions been answered?"]

After visiting with Mrs. P, I went to speak with Mrs. P's anesthesiologist to ask her about some specific processes and procedures that were used. ["What role do you play in the organization's process for a time out? How did you educate Mrs. P on the type of anesthesia that was used? Do you provide any specific guidance or help to patients with Mrs. P's particular issues and concerns?"]

I approached the operating room (OR) nurse and asked her a few questions about surgery and procedures in the OR used during Mrs. P's surgery. ["Can you describe the time-out process used in the OR during Mrs. P's surgery? What safety measures were used? When was your last emergency drill? Do you know what you can do in the event that you have a safety concern that you would like to report anonymously?"] I then reviewed the maintenance logs for the equipment used in the OR during Mrs. P's surgery, and spoke with the staff member responsible for the facility about her role. ["What is the center's process to main-

tain this equipment? How often is it checked? What is done with broken equipment or equipment in need of repair?"]

I proceeded to meet with center administrative staff to discuss any data or tracking of data relating to surgeries and postsurgical infections. As Infection Control had been one of the organization's priority focus areas, I opted to review this in relation to surgeries. ["What will you do to educate Mrs. P on postsurgical infection control and what she needs to tell the center if something develops? What if she develops an infection? Have you tracked postsurgical infection rates? How?"]

Later in the day, I took some time to discuss the case with the surgeon, asking her how she assessed and discussed the case with Mrs. P and what her process was for the surgical site marking and the time-out. I also asked about her process to prescribe medications, including if she used medication reconciliation information to determine what was prescribed postoperatively. ["What process was used for documenting your preoperative and postoperative notes? Describe the time-out process and your role. Has the center provided any information to you about unacceptable abbreviations, symbols, and acronyms? Did you use medication reconciliation information in your approach to medications and prescribing for Mrs. P? How was Mrs. P discharged from the surgical center?"] I then reviewed Mrs. P's discharge process by looking at notations in her medical record and interviewing the nurse involved in the discharge process. ["What was your role in discharging Mrs. P? What is the process for the surgeon to enter a postoperative note in the medical record? What education did you provide to Mrs. P and her family members before she left? What follow-up will typically take place after she leaves? Who is responsible for that?"]

Source: The Joint Commission: *Tracer Methodology: Tips and Strategies for Continuous Systems Improvement, 2nd Edition.* Oakbrook Terrace, IL: Joint Commission Resources, 2008; The Joint Commission: 2009 *Accreditation Process Guide for Ambulatory Care.* Oakbrook Terrace, IL: Joint Commission Resources, 2008.

the scan range.

— Ask patients with neurostimulators to shut them off temporarily while the scan is performed.

— Minimize x-ray exposure to the implanted or externally worn electronic medical device by using the lowest possible x-ray tube currently consistent with obtaining the required image quality and ensuring that the x-ray beam doesn't linger on the device for more than a few seconds.

■ When the CT procedure requires scanning for more than a few seconds over the device, medically trained staff should be ready to take emergency measures to treat any adverse reactions.

■ After scanning is complete, have the patient do the following:

— Turn the device back on if it was turned off before the scan.

— Check that the device works properly, even if the device was turned off.

— Contact his or her health care provider as soon as possible if he or she suspects that the device is not working properly.

Workflow Redesign

Workflow design is an important element of maintaining sterile conditions such as in the operating room or other clinical space. Improper or inconvenient space and flow design can affect sterile conditions, and can therefore lead to potentially increased risk of infection or error. An example is when the physical configuration of the space or work area does not provide for direct delivery of sterilized items to providers during a procedure.

Instances of how workflow can be affected by safety risks and environmental issues include the following[1]:

■ Delays of rescheduling because of equipment failure resulting from regular preventive maintenance

■ Examination cancellation because of poor screening by the physician, or failure to identify patient history or metal insertion in a previous surgical procedure

■ Risk identification associated with a lack of security measures around the site where a mobile imaging center is parked

---

TOOL: Just-in-Time and Kanban Cards

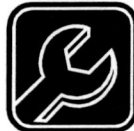

Just-in-time (JIT) is a strategy to control inventory and thus improve the return on investment of a business by reducing the associated carrying costs of overstocked inventory. The JIT philosophy is used in Lean thinking, based on the Toyota Production System.

To implement a JIT approach, a variety of systems need to be put in place. The most notable is a *kanban,* the Japanese word meaning "signal card." Using JIT and kanban cards is a wise business approach that ensures a continuous supply of inventory or product. A kanban is a visual control indicating it is time to replenish stock and perhaps reorder. Kanbans support the JIT philosophy. Kanban uses standard containers or lot sizes with a single card attached to each. Kanbans can be used for surgical kits, inventories, equipment, and forms. Kanban signals can include an empty bin, an alarm or alert, a light, or an outline painted on the floor.

A kanban should be inexpensive, be clear in its message, and elicit a rapid response. For instance, in a health care site's storage supply closet, the number of sterile gloves has fallen below a certain number. At that point a green line painted around the inside of the storage bin will be revealed. This green line indicates to the next staff member to come to that area that a requisition for more gloves must be made. This prevents the supply of gloves from dropping below a critical amount and allows care delivery to continue to flow smoothly. JIT is linked in concert with continuous improvement systems.

Kanbans work with JIT philosophy to prevent overstock and to smoothly replenish items on time, every time. Kanbans can be posted, painted, or labeled on a surface, including walls, ceilings, or floors. Colors, designs, and functions may be integrated to create a better functioning system. Kanbans can also be valuable in helping improve patient flow.

References

1. The Joint Commission: *Managing the Environment of Care in Ambulatory Care.* Oakbrook Terrace, IL: Joint Commission Resources, 2000.
2. Bifero A.E., Prakash J., Bergin J.: The role of chiropractic adjusting tables as reservoirs for microbial diseases. *Am J Infect Control* 34:155–157, Apr. 2006.
3. The Joint Commission: *Engaging Physicians in Patient Safety: A Handbook for Leaders.* Oakbrook Terrace, IL: Joint Commission Resources, 2006.
4. Agency for Healthcare Research and Quality, University of Michigan. AHRQ Healthcare Innovations Exchange. *Patient Safety Rounds Identify Systems Problems and Improve Perceptions of Commitment to Safety.* http://www.innovations.ahrq.gov/content.aspx?id=2261 (accessed Mar. 5, 2009).
5. The Joint Commission: *Applied Tracer Methodology: Tips and Strategies for Continuous Systems Improvement.* Oakbrook Terrace, IL: Joint Commission Resources, 2007.
6. The Joint Commission: *Safety in the Operating Room.* Oakbrook Terrace, IL: Joint Commission Resources, 2006.
7. Johnston J.: Toxic anterior segment syndrome—more than sterility meets the eye. *AORN J* 84:969–984, Dec. 2006.
8. The Joint Commission: *Steam Sterilization—Update on The Joint Commission's Position.* June 15, 2009. http://www.jointcommission.org/Library/WhatsNew/steam_sterilization.htm (accessed Sep. 1, 2009).
9. The Joint Commission:. Preventing accidents and injuries in the MRI suite. *Sentinel Event Alert 38,* Feb. 14, 2008. http://www.jointcommission.org/SentinelEvents/SentinelEventAlert/sea_38.htm (accessed Mar. 7, 2009).
10. Joint Commission Resources: Preventing infection in the MRI suite. *Environment of Care News* 12:8–9, Feb. 2009.
11. Conference of Radiation Control Program Directors. Inc.: *Image Gently™ Pediatric Campaign.* http://www.crcpd.org/CT/imagegently.html (accessed Feb. 23, 2009).
12. U.S Food and Drug Administration: FDA Preliminary Public Health Notification: Possible Malfunction of Electronic Medical Devices Caused by Computed Tomography (CT) Scanning. Jul. 14, 2008. http://www.fda.gov/cdrh/safety/071408-ctscanning.html (accessed May 12, 2009).

Chapter 7

STAFF EDUCATION AND TRAINING

Ambulatory staff training will involve some topics universal in health care and some topics particular to the ambulatory setting. Below are a few of those topics that have been shown in research to be of major importance for staff work with ambulatory patients. These include staff competency, orientation efforts, measures of a safety culture, specific in-service topics, and resources for training tools.

Competency

Patient safety depends on the alertness, mental acuity, and effectiveness of staff. Staff effectiveness is defined as the competency, skill mix, and number of staff in relation to the provisions of needed patient care.[1] Working in a smaller setting does not justify a relaxation of standards and qualifications.

When assigning a staff member to a particular team, role or responsibility, do not rely solely upon on-the-job training. Initial and ongoing competency assessment is an important part of maintaining patient safety. Skill mix matters—no matter how pressed you are, a clerk should not be asked to administer a medication. A full screening of the staff member's abilities, competencies and training background should be vetted.

Skill mix has a role to play in improving organizational effectiveness, and quality and safety of care, but competencies of individuals must be carefully assessed and documented. As an example, skill mix must be considered in point-of-care testing. Although point-of-care testing has improved turnaround time in many instances of patient care, rules must be adapted to ensure that test results are correct. These tests—which are performed upon specimens obtained from patients' bodies, such as blood, urine, cerebrospinal fluid, sputum, tissue, and so forth—represent variable risks to patients in ambulatory settings due to the possibility of false-positive or false-negative test results. Properly training staff to perform

these tests under adequate supervision enhances patient safety.

A "Sample Form for Competency Assessment," a useful tool that can be modified for your setting, is available at http://www.ormanager.com/toolbox.

Staff Orientation

Leadership has an obligation to inform and train each staff member regarding patient safety right from point of hire. Organizations must also determine each staff member's level of experience, knowledge, and skills related to patient safety (*see* the previous section, "Competency," in this chapter). However, training or experience does not equate with orienting this individual to the policies, required procedures, and expectations that your organization has established.

Orientation to the Organization and the Job

Patient safety should be a central tenet of health care provision in all organizations. Safety practices are the responsibility of all staff who encounter patients in the ambulatory environment. An organizational environment must be safe for patients to receive care, students and residents to learn, and providers to practice.

Although a multitude of standards, guidelines and policies are used or are available to be used for an organization's patient safety program, the clinical expertise for patient safety is developed through performance improvement projects and must be shared across the institution, with affiliated agencies and organizations, and at regional and national meetings. Staff should be oriented to the following:

- Current patient safety initiatives, including how staff are expected to participate
- The body of evidence behind these safety initiatives, to deepen staff members' understanding of the effects and risks in the care they are providing.

Figure 7-1. Safety Education Tool

Medication Safety Best Practices Guide

SAFETY EDUCATION	Level	Satisfactory
Prescribers and clinic staff are trained about appropriate procedures in the event of a serious medication error.	2	
All office staff, including physicians, physician assistants, nurse practitioners, nursing staff and office assistants attend educational programming on ways to avoid medication errors at least annually.	3	
The clinic staff received education about important drug safety issues on a regular basis as well as after a medication safety event or near-miss.	2	
New clinic staff underwent a period of training and evaluation of their knowledge, skills and performance prior to participating independently in patient care activities.	2	
Clinic staff received training on the proper use and maintenance of devices used in the clinic (e.g., glucose monitors, humidifiers, spacers used with inhalers, etc.) in a structured manner such as vendor presentation at the clinic or on-the-job training by a qualified clinic colleague.	2	
During orientation, clinic staff was taught strategies designed to reduce the risk of errors.	2	
When temporary agency staff was used, they have undergone appropriate training and orientation.	2	
Each staff member is assessed on skills and knowledge related to safe medication practices at least annually.	2	
The non-physicians are competent and well-trained for their jobs.	2	

This tool may be used to assess staff level of understanding for patient safety concerns.

Source: Creighton Health Services Research Program, Creighton University: *Medication Safety Best Practices Guide for Ambulatory Care Use.* http://chrp.creighton.edu/documents/bestpractices.pdf (accessed May 12, 2009). Permission given as open access.

- The particular organization's metrics for tracking and documenting data, specifically in ambulatory care
- The goals and objectives for eliminating medical errors and consequent medical injuries from clinical encounters and clinical practice

Staff should be encouraged to participate in healthy reporting practices. In an organization that nourishes a culture of safety, new staff are not only welcome to participate but contribute to growing the initiatives and the level of data.

Staff should also be encouraged to report and discuss near misses, as the related information may most quickly point to patient safety hot spots in a particular unit, department, or setting.

Another tool useful in assessing staff level of understanding for patient safety concerns is provided in Figure 7-1, above. Other tools for staff training and assessment are available from the Medical Group Management Association (*see* "Staff Training Tools" in this chapter, beginning on page 117, for more information).

Orientation to the Patient Safety Hot Spots

The Agency for Healthcare Research and Quality (AHRQ) has emphasized aspects of patient safety for which staff in a health care setting should receive orientation. AHRQ developed a four-element model for health care agencies to plan for patient safety. The four elements are listed in Table 7-1, page 107. Orient staff to patient safety hot spots using the AHRQ elements as a guide.

Table 7-1. Patient Safety Hot Spots	
AHRQ Patient Safety Elements	**Action Steps**
1. Identify threats to patient safety.	Move procedures and patients from surgical suites to ambulatory clinics.
2. Identify and evaluate effective patient safety practices.	Performance improvement team to review all procedures and identify safe and appropriate clinical settings for performance of procedures
3. Teach, disseminate, and implement effective patient safety practices.	Review of Joint Commission patient safety indicators and adapt them to develop your ambulatory procedure patient safety indicators. Include multiple education sessions of all involved in the care of patients undergoing ambulatory clinic procedures during the perioperative period.
4. Maintain vigilance.	Regularly review activities, monitoring compliance with policies for ambulatory clinic procedures, and infection control and surveillance. Periodically provide education through competency validation process and policy orientation to new employees, residents, faculty, and students.

Source: Modified from Kleinpeter M.A.: Standardizing ambulatory care procedures in a public hospital system to improve patient safety. In Henriksen K., et al. (eds.): *Advances in Patient Safety: From Research to Implementation.* Rockville, MD: Agency for Healthcare Research and Quality (AHRQ) and the Department of Defense Health Affairs. National Library of Medicine, 2004. http://www.ncbi.nlm.nih.gov/books/bv.fcgi?rid=aps.section.6867#6887 (accessed May 12, 2009).

How to Report Errors and Near Misses

An environment in which health care staff can report errors or potential errors (near misses or close calls) without fear of reprisal is the hallmark of a culture of safety.[2] Other highlights of a culture of safety in an organization include the following:

- Commitment to safety is one of the highest priorities of the organization.
- Necessary resources are provided by the organization.
- Safety is valued as the primary priority.
- Communication excellence among workers is encouraged.
- Unsafe acts are rare.
- There is openness about errors, and they are reported when they do occur.
- The response to a problem focuses on system improvement rather than individual blame.

The key—and the challenge—to fostering event and near-miss reporting is removing the fear of job loss, humiliation, and "shunning" by peers.[2] Disciplinary action is reserved for those instances that indicate willful disregard, wrongful intent, and noncompliance with reporting procedures. In turn, reporting is allotted some form

of recognition and acknowledgment. At Gundersen Lutheran Health System, each time a staff member reports an error, that person is sent a note of thanks and a small gift, such as package of LifeSavers→.[3] An event report is provided in Figure 7-2 (front and back), pages 108–109.

Staff should be given timely feedback on how the reported information was used, whether any changes for system-related improvement were made, or what plan of action—such as a root cause analysis or failure mode and effects analysis (FMEA)—will be implemented to make future changes.

For example, one military-based ambulatory care organization implemented an electronic communication process to inform staff about what happened as the result of a reported event and whether any processes were changed or enhanced as a result of the report.[2] Subsequently, the institution noted an 18% increase in the total number of errors reported over one year's time.

In two rural primary practices in New York State, a modified FMEA was used to anonymously survey staff

Figure 7-2. Medication Event Report

Date of Report

☐☐ / ☐☐ / ☐☐☐☐

Medication Event Report

Please report all events/incidents/errors you learn about - even those you find before they reach the patient. If you have questions on how to fill out this form, please contact your unit/department Medication Safety Liaison. If the event caused immediate harm or death, contact the Patient Safety Coordinator as soon as possible.

Patient's Name (Last, First with one letter per box)

☐☐☐☐☐☐☐☐☐☐☐☐☐☐☐☐☐☐☐☐☐☐☐☐☐☐☐☐☐☐

Medical Record Number

☐☐ - ☐☐ - ☐☐ - ☐

DOB

☐☐ / ☐☐ / ☐☐☐☐

Classification of the event: (check one)

_____ Near Miss

_____ Medication Error

_____ Adverse Drug Reaction - Non-Preventable

_____ IV Infiltrate of a Vesicant Drug

_____ Gross IV Infiltrate > 6 inches

Definitions:

Near Miss: A mistake in the medication process that is detected and corrected before actual medication administration.

Medication Error: A mistake in the medication process that was not caught and corrected before it reached the patient. Includes failure to use a medication.

ADR-non preventable: An unexpected reaction (not a side effect) to a drug that was used properly.   OR Dial 4 - A - D - R

The date the event occurred:

☐☐ / ☐☐ / ☐☐

Time of the event (use military time)

☐☐☐☐

Hospital Unit or Clinic Dept. / Location

☐☐☐☐☐

Describe the event and the patient outcome if known: (include such things as name of the medications involved, interventions taken, increased monitoring if needed, or difference between written order and what was given.)

Is there a change which could be made at Gundersen Lutheran which would prevent this event from occurring in the future?

Staff directly involved in the event: (circle all that apply)

| Nurse Anesthetist | Nurse, LPN | Medical Assistant | Pharmacist Technician | Physician Assistant | Other _____ |
| Nurse Practitioner | Nurse, Registered | Pharmacist | Physician | Unit Secretary / Clerk | |

Was physician notified of the event? ○ Yes   ○ No

Reporting Individual: (please circle)

Nurse   Physician   Pharmacist   Other _____

- -

This portion will be removed and sent back to you when information is complete. Thank you for reporting!

Name: (optional) _____

Dept. _____   Ext.: _____

STOP

After all information is recorded, send to unit / dept. Med Safety Liaison.

Figure 7-2. Medication Event Report (continued)

To be filled out by the unit / department Medication Safety Liaison. All forms should be sent to the Patient Safety Coordinator - Legal Department, immediately after review by the Medication Safety Liaison.

After reviewing the event information, check the type of error(s) involved. (Check all that apply)

____ Wrong dose ⟹ Dose ordered

Dose given

____ Wrong patient

____ Wrong time   Route ordered   Route given

____ Wrong route ⟹

____ Missed dose

____ Extra dose   Drug ordered   Drug given

____ Wrong drug ⟹

____ Wrong administration technique

____ Known allergy to drug

____ None of the Above

Other:_____

Stage in the medication process where the event first occurred: (Circle one)

Ordering / Prescribing   Transcription   Dispensing   Administration   Documentation   Monitoring   Discharge

Please assess the outcome of the reported event and check the appropriate severity level.
Note that medication events are defined as ADR's (adverse drug reactions, both preventable and non-preventable, medication errors, near misses and reported IV infiltrates.

____ Circumstances or events that have the capacity to result in an error. (No actual event occurred)

____ Event occurred but did not reach the patient (Doesn't include omissions)

____ Event occurred and reached the patient but did not cause patient harm. (Includes omissions)

____ Event occurred and reached patient which required monitoring to confirm it resulted in no harm to the patient and / or intervention to preclude harm

____ Event occurred that may have contributed to or resulted in temporary harm to patient and required intervention

____ Event occurred that may have contributed to or resulted in temporary harm to patient which required initial or prolonged hospitalization

____ Event occurred which may have contributed or resulted in permanent patient harm

____ Event occurred and required intervention necessary to sustain life

____ Event occurred and may have contributed to or resulted in patient's death

Date of liaison review

☐☐ / ☐☐ / ☐☐☐☐

Liaison's Name (Last, First with one letter per box)

☐☐☐☐☐☐☐☐☐☐☐☐☐☐☐☐☐☐☐☐☐☐☐☐☐☐☐☐☐☐☐

To be completed by Patient Safety Coordinator:

Tracking Number

Date scanned: _____   ☐☐☐☐☐☐☐☐☐

Source: Gundersen Lutheran Health System, La Crosse, WI: SCOPE Tool 5, Error Reporting, 2003. Used with permission.

on their perceptions of medical error frequency, severity, and cause.[4] Comparisons between staff groups (provider versus nursing versus administration) based on the top ten priorities perceived by staff, showed 53% agreement at one site and 30% at the other. Agreement between sites was 20%. The authors concluded that convergence of opinions within a practice is helpful to show that team members are "on the same page," but differing opinions should also be explored to help mutual understanding and foster teamwork. The advantage of employing a FMEA or another tool within practices is in revealing the specific issues faced in that setting and by that staff.

Another aspect of a culture of safety and an overriding patient safety program is a policy for disclosure of errors to patients. Experts increasingly predict that standard practice will be disclose, with apology and compensation, because it is not only the right thing to do but is a viable liability-claim-litigation avoidance strategy.[2] According to data from the Sorry Works! Coalition, mitigating a patient's anger over an error and resultant injury through disclosure will increase the number of settlements but will result in more justice for injured patients, fewer costly lawsuits and jury awards, and a reduction in defense costs.[2]

It is important to note that organization change experts claim it is not the official policies that drive organizations but rather the unwritten rules. For example, a clinical staff member skips a critical step in verifying a patient's identity and administers the wrong drug (one meant for another patient) because of time pressures in the clinic to increase patient throughput and keep on schedule.[5] Despite a policy calling for proper patient identification, patient safety is compromised here by virtue of the staff member's perception that production and efficiency are valued more by the clinic than compliance to safety procedures.

Measuring a Safety Culture

Using a safety culture survey in your organization can assess the climate for reporting. Many tools are available to assess the culture of safety. Researchers at the University of Texas have made their Safety Climate and Safety Attitudes Questionnaires available online for research purposes.[5,6] A simple, free registration form is requested. Particular tools for ambulatory settings are also available.

The survey is just the beginning step in the process

of improving patient safety. The real work, setting priorities for action and making changes, begins after communicating survey results to staff and managers. This helps to outline the topics for in-service training. Some of these topics may deal with the gap between attitudes and experiences, as described in the example above and patient identification procedures.

AHRQ also offers a culture survey for office-based settings. It is available for use at no charge and offers the opportunity to compare results with other sites (accessible at http://www.ahrq.gov/qual/patientsafetyculture/mosurvindex.htm).

Another helpful resource is the SCOPE toolkit from Gundersen Lutheran Health System, La Crosse, Wisconsin. Gundersen Lutheran is involved with 19 other medical centers in the Safety Collaborative for the OutPatient Environment (SCOPE), organized as a mini-collaborative of seven regional sites. Tools can be modified to suit a large, medium or small clinic.[7] The toolkit is available online at http://www.mch-hotlines.org/web/misc/scope.nsf.

Sexton et al. recommend taking the following steps to create and sustain a culture of safety[5]:
1. Assess the culture of safety.
2. Provide science-of-safety education to staff.
3. Identify safety concerns.
4. Establish senior leader partnerships with units.
5. Learn from one defect per month.
6. Reassess (remeasure) the culture of safety.

Specific In-Service/Training Topics

Some important topics for in-service include performance improvement, patient assessments (including the potential for falls), performing mobile lifts and transport safety, aseptic technique and sterilization monitoring, moderate sedation safety, fire safety, and communication and the development of effective teams (see also Chapter 2, "Communication").

Performance Improvement

Patient safety and performance improvement go hand in hand. Performance improvement projects and staff promote evidence-based best practices that improve patient safety, reduce risk, and prevent adverse incidents and sentinel events.

In November 2008 the Centers for Medicare & Medicaid Services (CMS) adopted the Hospital Outpatient Prospective Payment System final rule, which included revisions to the ambulatory surgical centers (ASCs) Conditions for Coverage (CfC), including changes to performance improvement requirements. In CfC 416.43, an ASC must develop, implement, and maintain an ongoing, data-driven quality assessment and performance improvement program that demonstrates measurable improvement in patient health outcomes and improves patient safety by using quality indicators or performance measures, and by the identification and reduction of medical errors. An ASC must also measure, analyze, and track quality indicators, adverse patient events, infection control, and other aspects of performance that includes care and services provided by the facility.[8]

Use of a performance improvement team process can involve all individuals in contact with the patient during an ambulatory procedure. Regardless of the research method you use, success will be assured if you do the following:

- Adopt a methodology to focus on injury prevention and reveal the risks.
- Study the problem at hand.
- Review all steps involved in each procedure.
- Develop a comprehensive procedure summary for all levels of care at the organization.
- Involve all stakeholders in the process to achieve buy-in and a willingness to adopt change.

There are a number of safety techniques and methods in the literature that can be selected to improve performance. The subject is too vast to cover in depth here. Much of this focuses on standardization of systems.

The primary objective of designing safe systems is to make it difficult for the individual to make an error. Standardization is integral in this. But because some errors inevitably occur, even with good systems, another aspect of any effective system must be to absorb these errors—that is, plan systems and processes to allow staff to detect errors. In this way, you are best facilitating their interception, as well as providing a means to mitigate consequences in cases where these potential errors are intercepted. The best systems take into account how people *should* react and respond (systemic factors) and how people *do* react and respond (human factors).

Training on Human Factors Engineering

Human factors engineering (HFE) encourages people to question when they identify red flags in any process or plan. Human factors, as a field of study, is the exploration of human abilities and characteristics as they affect the design and smooth operation of equipment, systems, and jobs. Human factors engineers and experts consider the strengths and weaknesses of human physical and mental abilities and how these affect a system's design. For example, it is now generally accepted that equipment such as ventilators, programmable IV pumps, and defibrillators are standardized in an inpatient setting. This illustrates the basic application of a human factors study. Wherever possible, equipment and procedure should be standardized to prevent veering off course and into risky territory.

HFE is an important component of any performance improvement imitative. HFE can be said to be the study of the interrelationships between humans, the tools they use, and the environment in which they live and work. HFE examines a particular activity in terms of its component tasks and then considers each task in terms of physical demands, skill demands, mental workload, and other such factors, along with their interactions with aspects of the work environment (such as adequate lighting, limited noise, or other distractions), device design, and team dynamics.

HFE has three components:

1. *Improve your philosophical, attitudinal view* that you're trying to redesign items—such as software, written text, architecture, devices–rather than working on people. There is a growing recognition that it is more effective, easier, makes more sense, and is less costly to fix the architecture, software, and so forth, than to remedy the actions of people. This is illustrated by the tongue-in-cheek comment: It is easier to bend metal than to twist arms.

2. *Understand the methods involved* when people are troubleshooting issues and equipment. The better your conceptual familiarity with your topic is, the better you will be able to discern why things are breaking or aren't working as they should or are not being used properly. You don't necessarily need to know how to use the equipment or process yourself, but you can ask the right questions to get the answers that will lead to a solution.

3. *Learn what HFE experts have found in terms of what*

Sidebar 7-1. The Timed Up and Go (TUG) Test

These are instructions for conducting the TUG test with a patient or client.

1. Equipment needed: arm chair, tape measure, tape, stop watch.

2. Begin the test with the patient sitting in a chair with arms. The patient's back should rest against the back of the chair. The chair should be stable and positioned such that it will not move when the patient moves from sitting to standing.

3. Place a piece of tape or other marker on the floor three meters away from the chair so that it is easily seen by the patient.

4. Instructions: "On the word *GO* you will stand up, walk to the line on the floor, turn around, and walk back to the chair and sit down. Walk at your regular pace."

5. Start timing on the word *"GO"* and stop timing when the patient is seated again correctly in the chair with his or her back resting on the back of the chair.

6. Patients should wear their regular footwear and may use any gait aid that they normally use during ambulation, but should not be assisted by another person. There is no time limit; do not rush the patient. They may stop and rest, standing, if needed.

7. Healthy older patients usually complete the task in 10 seconds or less. Very frail or weak elderly persons with poor mobility may take 2 minutes or more.

8. Give the patient a practice trial before giving a timed test.

9. Results correlate with gait speed, balance, functional level, and the ability to go out. Results can also change over time, and retesting should be done each year.

10. Interpretation
    - < 10 seconds = normal
    - < 20 seconds = good mobility, person can go out alone, mobile without a gait aid.
    - < 30 seconds = problems exist, person cannot go outside alone, requires a gait aid.

A score of more than or equal to 14 seconds has been shown to indicate a high risk of falls. Scores greater than 8.5 seconds are associated with high fall risk in community-dwelling older adults.

Sources: University of Pittsburgh Medical Center/Jefferson Regional Home Health, LP; Podsiadlo D., Richardson S.: The timed "Up & Go": a test of basic functional mobility for frail elderly persons. *J Am Geriatr Soc* 39:142–148, Feb. 1991; Shumway Cook A., Brauer S., Woollacott M.: Predicting the probability for falls in community dwelling older adults using the Timed Up & Go Test. Saskatoon Falls Prevention Consortium, Falls Screening and Referral Algorithm, TUG, Saskatoon Falls Prevention consortium, Jun. 2005. *Phys Ther* 80:896–903, Sep. 2000.

works and what doesn't in patient safety. For example, if you are investigating why providers override computer alerts on drug-drug interactions or written warnings in paper-based templates, HFE can help you understand the basis of their behavior in order to move forward in designing effective systems.

Patient Assessments

Choosing the right risk assessment tool, or a combination of tools, is important in maintaining the safety of patients. Risk assessment tools are generally of three categories: nursing fall risk assessments, functional assessments, and complete medical assessments.[1]

Nursing Fall Risk Assessments. Risk assessments typically provide a useful scale that predicts the likelihood of a patient fall. Examples of these types include the STRATIFY Risk Assessment Tool, the Reassessment is Safe Kare tool, the Morse Fall Scale, and the Hendrich Fall Risk Assessment tool.[1]

Proper patient assessment reduces the likelihood of injuries and deaths that result from falls.[9] Patient falls occur in all types of health care settings, but the issue of falls is increasing in ambulatory settings. Examples are patients falling after blood draws or falling off an imaging table in a radiation suite. Falls must also be considered, particularly in elderly or chronically ill patients, in ASCs. Joint Commission requirements call for reducing the risk of patient harm resulting from falls. Although to date, Joint Commission accreditation for ambulatory settings is not contingent on meeting this goal, the risks of falls in any setting are evident.

Assessment is key in meeting this goal. Any assessment that is undertaken must be *sensitive* (to correctly identify high-risk patients) and *specific* (to correctly identify patient not at risk).[1]

The first task in an assessment that is designed to ultimately prevent falls is to agree on a patient-fall definition. A number of useful and effective definitions selected by health care organizations are available in the literature.[1]

The next step in assessment is to correctly and completely evaluate a patient's risk of falling. Ambulatory care organizations can build this risk assessment into an initial assessment performed on the patient. Patient risk factors include the following:

- A history of previous falls
- Mental status
- Lack of or inadequate communication
- Sensory and auditory deficits (poor hearing or vision)
- Medications
- Urinary alternations
- Emotional upset

The University of Pittsburgh Medical Center (UPMC) Regional Home Health staff use the *Timed Up and Go* (TUG) test at the initial admission visit for home health services. This test is administered by a physical therapist to assess the patient's mobility. In physician practices and ambulatory centers, this test could be used with older adults and other specified patient populations to assess their risk of falling. The steps of a TUG test are presented in Sidebar 7-1, page 112.

Recognizing when an incident of falling has occurred, collecting and evaluating data, and designing a staff training activity for assessment techniques involves a commitment from the organization's leadership. The assessment is much more than just another piece of paperwork, but rather becomes the basis for clear communication with patients about their own risk for falls and a means to begin their own, and the family's, efforts to modify the home environment.

Functional Assessments. Functional assessments measure a patient's ability to manage daily routines of living. A functional assessment will help the provider assess the presence and severity of disease, a need for care, and change over time.[1] These techniques provide valuable information that can be used as the basis of preventive actions on the part of family, social work or related professionals, health care providers or agencies, or the patient him- or herself.

Comprehensive Medical Assessments. These assessments are used to predict falls in older adults. They can signal unmet medical needs and should send an alert for an in-depth diagnostic process and clinical intervention by a physician.

Environmental assessment is also important to overall patient safety. Occasional site surveys should identify falls hazards such as slippery floors, floors with wax buildup, cluttered areas, poor lighting, broken handrails or absence of handrails, and changes in floor grading, as well as the walking and running habits of staff, visitors, and patients.[1] Staff responsible for transporting patients should receive special preventive and adverse event reporting training in safety procedures.

Performing Mobile Lifts and Transport Safety

Use of mobile diagnostic (MRI, CT, or PET scans) and transport units is an area in which staff require special training in order to maintain safety for patients using the lift when entering an ambulatory clinic. The case study beginning on page 122 features safe practices used by an imaging company that encountered a number of risks to patient and staff safety.

Aseptic Technique and Sterilization Monitoring

Appropriate aseptic technique prepares patients for surgery and protects them from microorganisms in the environment and on the provider's skin, clothes, and hair; that is, it helps mitigate the risk of health care–acquired infections. Aseptic technique encompasses practices performed immediately before and during a surgical procedure. These include the following[10]:

- Handwashing (*see* Chapter 5, "Infection Prevention and Control")
- Surgical scrub
- Using surgical barriers, including sterile surgical drapes, and proper personal protective equipment, including head coverings, surgical masks and gowns, gloves, and shoe coverings
- Patient surgical prep
- Maintaining a sterile field
- Using safe operative techniques
- Maintaining a safe environment in the operating room

To provide comprehensive staff training in proper infection-prevention practices the organization should also do the following[10]:

- *Investigate to determine if proper aseptic technique is being followed* throughout the organization, particularly in areas where surgical procedures are performed, and if antiseptic products such as surgical scrubs and surface disinfectants are being used properly.
- *Hold regular in-service training* and provide updates on clinical/surgical infection-control techniques (*see* "Chapter 5, Infection Prevention and Control," and Chapter 6, "Environment and Equipment"). Staff are often confused about the differences between antiseptics and disinfectants and often use these solutions inappropriately. A comprehensive training program

includes the proper use of antiseptic solutions.

■ *Ensure that organization leaders serve as exemplary role models* for all personnel in proper infection control practices. Model aseptic behavior and encourage colleagues to do the same. When managers and leaders identify practices that endanger patients or staff, it is their obligation to address the improper behavior.

Moderate Sedation Safety

Nonanesthesiologist staff working with ambulatory anesthesia protocols must undergo assessment and receive adequate competency training. As the use of new agents such as propofol and fospropofol enter the menu of options for moderate sedation administration, the need for specific training is especially essential. (*See* Chapter 4, "Surgical Safety," for guidelines for training and useful tools.)

Fire Safety

Joint Commission requirements call for an organization to educate its staff, including licensed independent practitioners involved with surgical procedures, as well as anesthesia providers, regarding fire safety: controlling heat sources, managing fuels and attending to patient preparation, and establishing guidelines to minimize the oxygen concentration under drapes.

A comprehensive fire safety program involves creating objectives that are specified in planning and fully fleshed out in implementation. Objectives should include creating a multidisciplinary education program; creating guidelines for the safe use of devices via safety controls; and enabling the integration of knowledge with national guidelines. More details of a fire safety program are presented in Chapter 4, "Surgical Safety," page 61.

Teamwork (Building Effective Teams)

Providing safe health care depends on highly trained individuals with disparate roles and responsibilities acting together in the best interests of the patient. Communication barriers across hierarchies, failure to acknowledge human fallibility, and lack of situational awareness combine to cause poor teamwork, which can lead to clinical adverse events. Effective teamwork and communication are associated with better patient outcomes, higher patient satisfaction, and greater patient safety.

Common teamwork barriers are listed in Table 7-2, above.

Table 7-2. Common Barriers to Effective Teamwork

- Inconsistency in team leaders
- Lack of time to meet and interact as a team
- Hierarchy
- Defensiveness
- Not speaking up
- Conventional thinking
- Varying communication styles
- Unresolved conflict
- Distractions
- Fatigue
- Heavy workload
- Misinterpreting cues
- Lack of role clarity

Source: Agency for Healthcare Research and Quality (AHRQ) and the Department of Defense (DoD): Team-STEPPS™ Tools and Materials, 2009.

According to the Canadian Patient Safety Institute, health care teamwork is based on sufficient knowledge, skills, and attitudes.[11] Sidebar 7-2, page 115, presents a list of what those baseline attributes should be.

Some of Kaiser Permanente's project efforts to improve teamwork include assertiveness training, briefing and debriefing procedures, communication skills, and situational awareness.[5] Their rationale is as follows:

■ Assertiveness training empowers staff to speak up and "stop the line" when they have a safety concern.
■ Briefings are communications between team members that provide a time to raise concerns, clarify a plan of care, and relay important information either before a procedure begins or after an event occurs.
■ Situational awareness raises awareness of what is going on around you to decrease risks of errors.

For training in communication, many organizations use the SBAR technique to synchronize the style of the communication they employ. SBAR stands for Situation, Background, Assessment, and Recommendation. This method, devised to help bridge the gap between the way clinical staff and physicians are taught to communicate, has been found to be one of the fastest ways to communicate information in a manner that is efficient and to the point.[5]

■ **S:** Define the problem (situation).
■ **B:** Keep information brief, related, and to the point (background).

Sidebar 7-2. Knowledge, Skills, and Attitudes That Promote Teamwork

Knowledge

Health care professionals who work effectively in teams for patient safety understand the following:

- The roles and responsibilities of each team member, including decision making, supervision and support, and the expectations and requirements for individual performance
- The skills, competencies, experience and scopes of practice of team members, including overlaps and gaps in the team's capabilities
- Team dynamics and authority gradients, and the importance of relevant expertise as a basis for leadership in a given situation
- A shared vocabulary to facilitate effective communication within the team
- Key safety issues and priorities inherent in team practice and pertinent to the patient population served
- Protocols for the team's response to adverse events, including appropriate disclosure to patients, debriefing, and team support
- The impact of technology on team dynamics
- How to use evidence-informed team communication tools to facilitate the improvement of patient safety, including: permission and invitation to speak up, question, and challenge; conversational turn-taking; listening; checklists and briefing
- How to give transparent feedback that fosters team development
- How to provide appropriate debriefing and team support after an adverse event or close call
- How to monitor and evaluate team performance
- The rationale for and implementation of team processes, policies, and procedures
- The resources and administrative skills required to achieve the team's objectives for patient care
- The team's role within the health care system
- How to proactively address concerns about provider or system performance involving risk to patients and/or team members through the appropriate channels

Skills

Health care professionals who work effectively in teams for patient safety do the following:

- Manage and prevent conflict, and conduct effective negotiations
- Apply standardized team processes and protocols to ensure reliability and shared understanding
- Use appropriate shared clinical documentation to facilitate continuity of care
- Exercise decision-making authority in a situation-appropriate manner
- Set clear parameters for independent decision making
- Provide consultation, delegation, and support, and delegate tasks as appropriate

Attitudes

Health care professionals who work effectively in teams for patient safety do the following:

- Demonstrate respect and professionalism
- Are committed to fulfilling their individual responsibilities in the team environment
- Are receptive to constructive feedback about care, and provide constructive feedback to others
- Participate in shared interprofessional team learning, including setting measurable team goals and priorities, and in implementing continuous quality improvement
- Accept the team as an evidence-informed community of practice for learning
- Foster an environment in which the team works to provide the best possible patient outcomes
- Foster an environment in which each member of the team both learns from and teaches other team members
- Foster an environment in which responsibility for care and accountability for outcomes is appropriately shared, such that each individual in a team is held accountable for the quality of his or her work
- Practice patient-centered care such that the patient and family are visibly active team participants
- Facilitate continuity of care (through integrated, interprofessional, individualized care plans that extend across the organization and across all care transitions and that belong to the patient)
- Advocate for individual patients and for appropriate resources to meet their needs

Source: Frank J.R., Brien S. (eds.) The Safety Competencies Steering Committee: *The Safety Competencies: Enhancing Patient Safety Across the Health Professions.* Ottawa, ON: Canadian Patient Safety Institute, 2008.

Table 7-3. Joint Commission Suggested Actions to Address Disruptive Behavior

1. Educate all team members—both physicians and nonphysician staff—on appropriate professional behavior defined by the organization's code of conduct. The code and education should emphasize respect. Include training in basic business etiquette (particularly phone skills) and people skills.[1–3]

2. Hold all team members accountable for modeling desirable behaviors, and enforce the code consistently and equitably among all staff regardless of seniority or clinical discipline in a positive fashion through reinforcement as well as punishment.[1,4–7]

3. Develop and implement policies and procedures/ processes appropriate for the organization that address the following:
   —"Zero tolerance" for intimidating and/or disruptive behaviors, particularly the most egregious instances of disruptive behavior such as assault and other criminal acts. Incorporate the zero tolerance policy into medical staff bylaws and employment agreements as well as administrative policies.
   —Medical staff policies regarding intimidating and/or disruptive behaviors of physicians within a health care organization should be complementary and supportive of the policies that are present in the organization for nonphysician staff.
   —Reducing fear of intimidation or retribution and protecting those who report or cooperate in the investigation of intimidating, disruptive and other unprofessional behavior.[1,2] Nonretaliation clauses should be included in all policy statements that address disruptive behaviors.
   —Responding to patients and/or their families who are involved in or witness intimidating and/or disruptive behaviors. The response should include hearing and empathizing with their concerns, thanking them for sharing those concerns, and apologizing.[7]
   —How and when to begin disciplinary actions (such as suspension, termination, loss of clinical privileges, reports to professional licensure bodies)

4. Develop an organization process for addressing intimidating and disruptive behaviors (LD.03.01.01, EP 5) that solicits and integrates substantial input from an interprofessional team, including representation of medical and nursing staff, administrators, and other employees.[1,2,5]

5. Provide skills-based training and coaching for all leaders and managers in relationship-building and collaborative practice, including skills for giving feedback on unprofessional behavior, and conflict resolution.[1,5,7–10] Cultural assessment tools can also be used to measure whether or not attitudes change over time.

6. Develop and implement a system for assessing staff perceptions of the seriousness and extent of instances of unprofessional behaviors and the risk of harm to patients.[1,2,9]

7. Develop and implement a reporting/surveillance system (possibly anonymous) for detecting unprofessional behavior. Include ombuds services[10] and patient advocates,[4,7] both of which provide important feedback from patients and families who may experience intimidating or disruptive behavior from health care professionals. Monitor system effectiveness through regular surveys, focus groups, peer and team member evaluations, or other methods.[1] Have multiple and specific strategies to learn whether intimidating or disruptive behaviors exist or recur, such as through direct inquiries at routine intervals with staff, supervisors, and peers.

8. Support surveillance with tiered, nonconfrontational interventional strategies, starting with informal "cup of coffee" conversations directly addressing the problem and moving toward detailed action plans and progressive discipline, if patterns persist.[1,5,7,11] These interventions should initially be nonadversarial in nature, with the focus on building trust, placing accountability on and rehabilitating the offending individual, and protecting patient safety.[5,11] Make use of mediators and conflict coaches when professional dispute resolution skills are needed.[5,8,12]

9. Conduct all interventions within the context of an organization commitment to the health and well-being of all staff,[7] with adequate resources to support individuals whose behavior is caused or influenced by physical or mental health pathologies.

10. Encourage interprofessional dialogues across a variety of forums as a proactive way of addressing ongoing conflicts, overcoming them, and moving forward through improved collaboration and communication.[1,4,5,13]

11. Document all attempts to address intimidating and disruptive behaviors.[2]

References

1. Porto G., Lauve R.: Disruptive clinical behavior: A persistent threat to patient safety. *Patient Safety and Quality Healthcare*, Jul.–Aug. 2006. Available online: http://www.psqh.com/julaug06/disruptive.html (accessed Apr. 14, 2008).

2. ECRI Institute: Disruptive practitioner behavior report, Jun. 2006. Available for purchase online: http://www.ecri.org/Press/Pages/Free_Report_Behavior.aspx (accessed Apr. 14, 2008)

3. Kahn M.W.: Etiquette-based medicine. *N Engl J Med*, 358:1988–1989, May 8, 2008.

> ## Table 7-3. Joint Commission Suggested Actions to Address Disruptive Behavior (continued)
>
> 4. Institute for Safe Medication Practices: Survey on work-place intimidation. 2003. Available online: https://ismp.org/Survey/surveyresults/Survey0311.asp (accessed Apr. 14, 2008)
> 5. Gerardi D.: Effective strategies for addressing "disruptive" behavior: Moving from avoidance to engagement. Medical Group Management Association Webcast, 2007; and, Gerardi, D: Creating Cultures of Engagement: Effective Strategies for Addressing Conflict and "Disruptive" Behavior. Arizona Hospital Association Annual Patient Safety Forum, 2008
> 6. Leape L.L., Fromson J.A.: Problem doctors: Is there a system-level solution? *Ann Intern Med* 144:107–155, 2006.
> 7. Hickson G.B.: A complementary approach to promoting professionalism: Identifying, measuring, and addressing unprofessional behaviors. *Acad Med* 82:1040–1048, Nov. 2007.
> 8. Gerardi D.: The emerging culture of health care: Improving end-of-life care through collaboration and conflict en-
>
> gagement among health care professionals. *Ohio State Journal on Dispute Resolution* 23(1):105–142, 2007.
> 9. Keogh T., Martin, W.: Managing unmanageable physicians. *Physician Exec* 18–22, Sep.–Oct. 2004.
> 10. Marshall P., and Robson R.: Preventing and managing conflict: Vital pieces in the patient safety puzzle. *Healthc Q* 8:39–44, Oct. 2005.
> 11. Ransom S.B., et al.: Enhancing physician performance. American College of Physician Executives, Tampa, Fla., chapter 4, pp. 45–72, 2000.
> 12. Hickson G.B., et al; Patient complaints and malpractice risk in a regional healthcare center. *South Med J* 100:791–796, Aug. 2007.
> 13. Rosenstein A.H., O'Daniel M.: Disruptive behavior and clinical outcomes: Perceptions of nurses and physicians. *Am J Nurs* 105:1,54–64, 2005.
>
> **Source:** The Joint Commission: Behaviors that undermine a culture of safety. *Sentinel Event Alert* #40. Oakbrook Terrace, IL: The Joint Commission. Jul. 9, 2008.

- **A:** Summarize what you found/think (assessment).
- **R:** Describe what you want (recommendation).

The Institute for Healthcare Improvement Web site at http://www.ihi.org explains in detail how to carry out the SBAR technique. As an example, when a health system in the Midwest learned from their staff assessments that many respondents lacked training in formal error prevention techniques (20%), training in error reporting (30%), and awareness of common errors occurring in their facilities (49%), they developed four training modules on the topics of safety culture, caregiver communication, human factors, and knowledge of reporting. The health system used a train-the-trainer format and deployed toolkits comprising slide presentations and overheads, instructor guides, unit posters, quick-reference cards, and postprogram tests.[5]

Disruptive behavior among health care workers has reached the point that The Joint Commission saw fit to issue a *Sentinel Event Alert* on this issue, and a new Leadership standard requires an organization to have a code of conduct that defines acceptable and disruptive and inappropriate behaviors. A list of suggested actions appears in Table 7-3, beginning on page 116. This has to be one of the most difficult areas of an organization's culture to address, particularly in institutions where the major disrupter is also a major revenue source and/or well connected politically.

Staff Training Tools

A number of useful tools are available online. A few of them are mentioned below.

The Health Research and Educational Trust, the Institute for Safe Medication Practices, and the Medical Group Management Association offers the *Physician Practice Patient Safety Assessment*®, a self-assessment tool that helps physician practices evaluate their patient-safety processes and detect areas for improvement. In 2009 the partners released *Pathways for Patient Safety*™, a series of Web-based modules aimed at increasing awareness, knowledge, and implementation of best practices to reduce the risk of patient harm in physician practices. The three modules (teamwork, patient assessment, and medication safety) are all downloadable, with free registration, at http://www.mgma.com/solutions or http://www.pathwaysforpatientsafety.org.[12]

AHRQ and the Department of Defense (DoD) have conducted research on high-stress, high-risk and complex work environments including the field of medicine.[13] They have synthesized their findings into a set of free, easily accessible teamwork and communication tools called Team-STEPPS™. The toolkit is an evidence-based teamwork system aimed at optimizing patient outcomes by improving communication and other teamwork skills among health care professionals. The TeamSTEPPS™ program is available free of charge at the AHRQ Web site at http://www.ahrq.gov/

Figure 7-3. TeamSTEPPS™ Teamwork Attitudes Questionnaire (T-TAQ)

Please complete the following questionnaire by placing a check mark [√] in the box that corresponds to your level of agreement from *Strongly Disagree* to *Strongly Agree*. Answer every question and select only one response for each question. The questionnaire is anonymous, so please do not put your name or any other identifying information on the questionnaire.

[Optional]: On the last page you will find questions about your background and experience. Please provide your responses to each question in the space provided. Thank you for your participation.

TeamSTEPPS

TeamSTEPPS™ Teamwork Attitudes Questionnaire

The purpose of this survey is to measure your impressions of various components of teamwork as it relates to patient care and safety.

Instructions: Please respond to the questions below by placing a check mark (√) in the box that corresponds to your level of agreement from *Strongly Disagree* to *Strongly Agree*. Please select only one response for each question.

		Strongly Disagree	Disagree	Neutral	Agree	Strongly Agree
Team Structure						
1.	It is important to ask patients and their families for feedback regarding patient care.					
2.	Patients are a critical component of the care team.					
3.	This facility's administration influences the success of direct care teams.					
4.	A team's mission is of greater value than the goals of individual team members.					
5.	Effective team members can anticipate the needs of other team members.					
6.	High-performing teams in health care share common characteristics with high-performing teams in other industries.					
Leadership						
7.	It is important for leaders to share information with team members.					
8.	Leaders should create informal opportunities for team members to share information.					
9.	Effective leaders view honest mistakes as meaningful learning opportunities.					
10.	It is a leader's responsibility to model appropriate team behavior.					
11.	It is important for leaders to take time to discuss with their team members plans for each patient.					
12.	Team leaders should ensure that team members help each other out when necessary.					

PLEASE CONTINUE TO THE NEXT PAGE ⟹

American Institutes for Research®   Version 1.0, July 2008   Page 1 of 3

Before staff completes the questionnaire, read the initial instructions aloud.

Figure 7-3. TeamSTEPPS™ Teamwork Attitudes Questionnaire (T-TAQ) (continued)

TeamSTEPPS

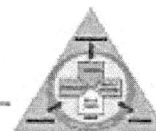

		Strongly Disagree	Disagree	Neutral	Agree	Strongly Agree
Situation Monitoring						
13.	Individuals can be taught how to scan the environment for important situational cues.					
14.	Monitoring patients provides an important contribution to effective team performance.					
15.	Even individuals who are not part of the direct care team should be encouraged to scan for and report changes in patient status.					
16.	It is important to monitor the emotional and physical status of other team members.					
17.	It is appropriate for one team member to offer assistance to another who may be too tired or stressed to perform a task.					
18.	Team members who monitor their emotional and physical status on the job are more effective.					
Mutual Support						
19.	To be effective, team members should understand the work of their fellow team members.					
20.	Asking for assistance from a team member is a sign that an individual does not know how to do his/her job effectively.					
21.	Providing assistance to team members is a sign that an individual does not have enough work to do.					
22.	Offering to help a fellow team member with his/her individual work tasks is an effective tool for improving team performance.					
23.	It is appropriate to continue to assert a patient safety concern until you are certain that it has been heard.					
24.	Personal conflicts between team members do not affect patient safety.					

PLEASE CONTINUE TO THE NEXT PAGE ⟹

American Institutes for Research®   Version 1.0, July 2008   Page 2 of 3

((continued on page 120))

119

**Figure 7-3. TeamSTEPPS™ Teamwork Attitudes Questionnaire (T-TAQ)
(continued)**

Communication	Strongly Disagree	Disagree	Neutral	Agree	Strongly Agree
25. Teams that do not communicate effectively significantly increase their risk of committing errors.					
26. Poor communication is the most common cause of reported errors.					
27. Adverse events may be reduced by maintaining an information exchange with patients and their families.					
28. I prefer to work with team members who ask questions about information I provide.					
29. It is important to have a standardized method for sharing information when handing off patients.					
30. It is nearly impossible to train individuals how to be better communicators.					

Please provide any additional comments in the space below.

Thank you for your participation!

Source: TeamSTEPPS™ Tools and Materials, 2009.

teamstepps or the Department of Defense Patient Safety Program Web site at http://dodpatientsafety.usuhs.mil/teamstepps.

One component of TeamSTEPPS™ is the Teamwork Attitudes Questionnaire (T-TAQ), presented in Figure 7-3, beginning on page 118, which can be used to assess the level of quality of teamwork in your organization and the specific needs within a unit or group.

References

1. The Joint Commission: *Good Practices in Preventing Patient Falls: A Collection of Case Studies.* Oakbrook Terrace, IL: Joint Commission Resources, 2007.
2. Cited in Shostek K.: Developing a culture of safety in ambulatory settings. *J Ambul Care Manage* 30:105–113, Apr.–Jun. 2007.
3. Schauberger C., et al.: Gundersen Lutheran Health System, Ambulatory Patient Safety Toolkit. Safety Collaborative for the OutPatient Environment (SCOPE), 2002. http://www.gundluth.org/?id=846&sid=1 (accessed Feb. 9, 2009).
4. Singh R., et al.: Prioritizing threats to patient safety in rural primary care. *J Rural Health* 23:173–178, Mar. 28, 2007.
5. Sexton J.B., Thomas E.J.: *The Safety Climate Survey: Psychometric and Benchmarking Properties.* Technical Report 03-03. The University of Texas Center of Excellence for Patient Safety Research and Practice (AHRQ grant # 1PO1HS1154401 and U18HS1116401), 2003. http://www.uth.tmc.edu/schools/med/imed/patient_safety/survey&tools.htm (accessed May 15, 2009).
6. Sexton J.B., et al.: The Safety Attitudes Questionnaire: Psychometric Properties, Benchmarking Data, and Emerging Research. *BMC Health Services Research* 6:44, Apr. 3, 2006. http://www.biomedcentral.com/ 1472-6963/6/44/abstract (accessed May 15, 2009).
7. Gundersen Lutheran Health System: *Ambulatory Patient Safety Toolkit. Safety Collaborative for the OutPatient Environment (SCOPE).* http://www.gundluth.org (accessed Feb. 9, 2009).
8. Pyrek K.M.: ASCs still digesting new CfCs. *SurgiStrategies* 7/2/09, http://www.surgistrategies.com/articles/new-medicare-cfcs-for-ascs.html (accessed Jul. 20, 2009).
9. The Joint Commission: *Engaging Physicians in Patient Safety: A Handbook for Leaders.* Oakbrook Terrace, IL: Joint Commission Resources, 2006.
10. *Infection Control Today:* Practice for perioperative nurses: aseptic technique and the sterile field, Apr. 1, 2005. http://www.infectioncontroltoday.com/articles/541feat1.html. (accessed Mar. 8, 2009).
11. Frank J.R., Brien S. (eds): *The Safety Competencies Steering Committee: The Safety Competencies: Enhancing Patient Safety Across the Health Professions.* Ottawa, Ontario: Canadian Patient Safety Institute, 2008.
12. Pathways for Patient Safety: Health Research and Educational Trust, Institute for Safe Medication Practices, Medical Group Management Association, 2009. http://www.mgma.com or http://www.pathwaysforpatientsafety.org (accessed May 15, 2009).
13. Agency for Healthcare Research and Quality (AHRQ); U.S. Department of Defense (DoD): *TeamSTEPPS™ Tools and Materials.* 2009. http://teamstepps.ahrq.gov/abouttoolsmaterials.htm. (accessed May 15, 2009).

Case Study: Lift Safety

CASE STUDY AT A GLANCE

Name: INSIGHT IMAGING

Setting: Ambulatory, diagnostic imaging services

Patient safety topic: Lift safety for mobile diagnostic imaging

Accomplishment: Succeeded in reaching 100% lift safety goal and to eliminate 100% of "near miss" accidents

The Organization

INSIGHT IMAGING is a provider of diagnostic imaging services, through a network of fixed-site centers and mobile facilities. Company headquarters are located in Lake Forest, California. The company provides services around the country, with emphasis on their targeted regional markets, which include California, Arizona, New England, The Carolinas, Florida, and the Mid-Atlantic states.

Services include magnetic resonance imaging (MRI), computerized tomography (CT), and positron emission tomography (PET) and combined PET/CT. INSIGHT serves more than 600,000 patients nationwide on an annual basis through a network of approximately 60 fixed-site imaging centers and 100 mobile diagnostic imaging units. The fixed sites also offer radiography (x-ray), fluoroscopy, mammography, ultrasound, bone densitometry, and radiation therapy. The highly trained staff consists of radiologists, technologists, nurses, assistants, clerical staff, and a staff of experienced transportation fleet members.

Project Beginnings
Project Name and Goals
In 2004 the INSIGHT IMAGING quality improvement team looked for upcoming performance improvements in the mobile division that were unique to its environment. The quality team looked at occurrence data, staff input, and risk management information from across the country. A potential risk was identified on the lift of the mobile unit. This lift transports patients into and off of the mobile unit. The identified risk put in jeopardy not only patients but also staff.

The team reviewed benchmarking standards, compared occurrences with other companies that had mobile units with lifts, spoke to the manufacturers of the lifts, and most importantly, spoke to the staff that use the mobile units every day. This performance improvement was identified as high importance, high risk, and high volume in that 100% of their patients use the lift.

Interestingly enough, they found that the staff had many "near miss" episodes of potential risk. The near-miss accidents concerned incidents when staff almost fell off the unit after they assumed that the lift was up when the door was opened. The team looked at risks of accidental tripping over rugs as well, and later rugs were replaced due to this hazard. Staff had also been telling patients not to lean on the movable part of the lift, but were leaning on it themselves. If this was witnessed, it was written as a "near miss," meaning that they had the potential to fall off the lift. Some employees were so comfortable going up and down the lift that they didn't hold on any longer. The team counted this as a "near miss" too. Near misses were recorded and the employee was reeducated to the safety elements that were implemented.

The team looked at this as a process and prioritized what they were going to do by the importance of reducing risk to staff and patients. Staff conduct constant improvement in their process to make it safer for staff and patients. Though they have been able to make lift accidents and near accidents a thing of the past, they are ever-vigilant for future safety and compliance of staff.

Needs Identification and Baseline Measures
Benchmarking for ambulatory health care is weak, and in mobile imaging, it is nonexistent. Therefore, the team spoke with quality managers at two mobile companies who agreed with the data that had been collected. They also looked at five years of data within the company and at accounts of accidents of other mobile companies. These companies were aware that both the measurements used and the resulting data were poor

Case Study: Lift Safety (continued)

Team Members and Roles

The performance improvement team consisted of a regional vice president, managers, technologists, aides, nurses, risk management, the quality improvement director (team leader), and fleet members. Fleet members are the employees who drive and maintain the mobile units. They set up for the day after transporting the mobile unit and secure it for moving it at the end of the day. Fleet members work closely with the technologists. The team addressed the issues on a monthly basis with all of the operations managers.

Project Activity

Project Steps

As the team prioritized its process for risk reduction, it became clear what needed to be done. The steps were to do the following:

1. Look at the safety features that came with the mobile lifts and investigate whether staff were using them as they were designed.
2. Make any modifications to the lift to reduce risk.
3. Evaluate that the modifications worked.

This was anticipated as being a simple improvement process. However, it soon became more complicated and the team was led to better refine the improvement process.

As the safety features were reviewed, it became clear that the lift locks that came from the manufacturers were not intended to have someone lean on them. Patients and staff who leaned on the movable part of the gate had the potential to fall off the lift. The lift is about six feet off the ground.

The second identified problem was that the lift was usually in the down position. If someone opened the lift door, the lift may have been in the down position creating an immediate six-foot drop.

These were identified as changes that needed to be made. In the mobile business, making a change to any location is challenging. The units and staff are spread throughout the country; thus making a change throughout the mobile environment means communication must take place with hundreds of staff who are constantly on the move throughout many states.

The changes to be made were to do the following:
1. Put safety locks on the movable part of the gate.
2. Teach staff that the lift must remain in the up position if anyone is on board. All staff education is done via conference calls, small-group meetings, and e-mail communication. The team also created an employee checklist for self-evaluation, which helps the employee remember what the changes are until it becomes routine.

After installation of the locks and staff training was implemented, a random sampling of site compliance was done. The results were good, but not great. Although the team had hit its compliance goal, it found that staff had the security of believing that the safety locks would hold them if they leaned on them. Staff went back to the safety team to see what they could add to lift safety.

A fleet member came up with the idea that the safety lock and side rails on the movable sides should be flagged with a warning. The signage was ordered and stickers were placed on the safety lock and movable side rails. The safety lock stated, "Lock should be closed before moving," and the side rails stated, "Do not hold or lean on rails." After those were deployed and educational in-services were given, the evaluation team randomly sampled compliance.

Although they hit their new target, the reviewers were still not satisfied that they had done everything that they could to reduce risk. They went back to the team. The team put together an educational slide presentation to send to all staff as a reminder of lift safety compliance. Because many of their mobile units are in very rural and remote areas, this was not a valuable tool across the board. Many sites were not able to use it.

(continued on page 124)

Case Study: Lift Safety (continued)

Again, the reviewers went back to the team. The fleet members conceived of an idea to ensure that their patients stood in a safe location on the lift. A square block or footprints were painted on the lift to mark EX-ACTLY where the patient was to stand. Tape marks or padding were placed on the nonmovable part of the rail where they were to hold on. Staff was educated about the newest changes and evaluated results. At the end of 2007, they had made the changes that they could to provide a safe environment for staff and patients. Their only remaining concern was and still continues to be staff compliance.

Because they had reduced "near misses" and any occurrences, the team was concerned about compliance with all of the changes. A continuous compliance worksheet was designed and included in the evaluation of every employee in 2008. The continuous compliance worksheet has helped remind staff and managers to look for lift safety compliance (Figure 7-4, page 125).

The Tools Used

The team performed a literature search from two leading MRI researchers, but nothing was available to assist in safety practices for mobile MRI. The team devised a tool to track continuous compliance, presented in Figure 7-4.

Old Process/Plan vs. New

In the old process, there was no policy to follow, no compliance tracking, and no visual signals (kanbans) to assist maintenance of safe practices. In the new processes, these exist (*see* Figures 7-5, 7-6, and 7-7 on page 126) in the form of markings and colors on stairs, warning and reminder signs, and other visual positioning cues.

Staff Training and Education

Because the mobile staff are located across the country, they used online PowerPoint presentations and conference calls, and the area and operations managers had direct contact with the staff for education and compliance.

The Outcome

Measurable Outcomes

The team measured outcomes by means of compliance tools, specifically the continuous compliance worksheet shown in Figure 7-4, page 125.

Lessons Learned

The undertaking was more difficult than first anticipated because the lift safety team continued to find ways to improve the process. The team reports that it will probably never let this one rest, as errors with lifts have the potential to be catastrophic.

The lessons learned in this project that will continue in future projects are that staff input, multi-modality team input, and staff compliance are the critical pieces to making performance improvements successful. INSIGHT no longer has *any* patients or staff members falling off the lift and hurting themselves.

Case Study: Lift Safety (continued)

Figure 7-4. Mobile Continuous Compliance Checklist

INSIGHT
IMAGING
Results. Right. Now.

Mobile Continuous Compliance Checklist

SITE/FACILITY: _____

EMPLOYEE: _____ DATE: _____

	YES	NO
1. Lift is in the up position.	____	____
2. Daily log is completed.	____	____
If not, why _____		
3. Each employee is wearing a name badge	____	____
4. The 2nd patient identifier was used by each employee.	____	____
5. The lift control device is easily reached from the street level when the lift is in the up position.	____	____
6. Employees are washing their hands every time they cross the scan room threshold.	____	____
7. Employees are using gloves for inserting and removing IV's.	____	____
8. IV discharge instructions were given to all patients.	____	____
9. Employees are assisting patient on and off the table.	____	____
10. Coils are wiped down after every patient.	____	____
11. A medication sheet is created for every patient receiving contrast.	____	____
12. Each patient is offered to take a medication sheet home.	____	____
13. The tech has reviewed all areas of the assessment sheet with the patient and signs it.	____	____
14. All syringes are labeled.	____	____
15. Pillows are not placed on the footrest.	____	____
16. No needle is recapped.	____	____
17. Patient is holding non-moveable railing when lift is moving.	____	____
18. Sharps container is not ¾ full or more.	____	____
19. Dirty laundry is held away from body.	____	____
20. Correct ergonomics is being used.	____	____
21. Each patient is being asked if they have any special needs such as hearing, visual or cultural needs.	____	____
22. Each patient is being asked if they have pain.	____	____
23. Each patient is being asked what can be done to make them feel more comfortable.	____	____
24. The technologist asks each patient receiving contrast about renal (kidney problems) disease, dialysis and diabetes.	____	____
25. The medication reconciliation sheet is being checked off on a monthly basis. This record includes all drugs given on the unit.	____	____

Manager's Signature   Date

_____   _____

Use of the checklist helps quality and safety experts ensure that compliance is followed. This list is continually being updated and refined.

Source: INSIGHT IMAGING, Lake Forest, CA.

(continued on page 126)

Case Study: Lift Safety (continued)

Figure 7-5. Visual Cues: Warnings

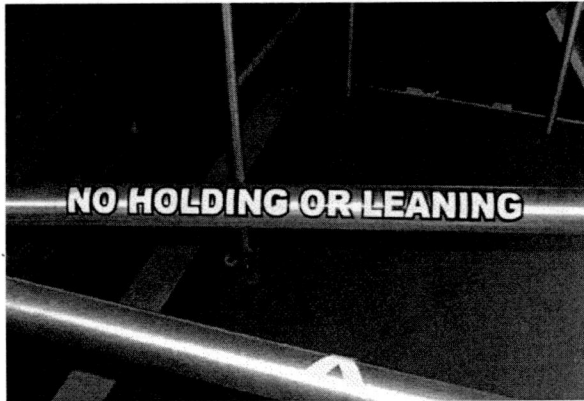

Warning signs signal patients to keep away from the rails.

Source: INSIGHT IMAGING, Lake Forest, CA.

Figure 7-6. Visual Cues: Signage

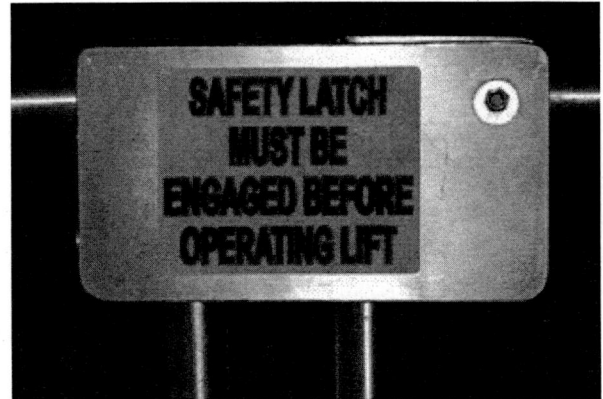

A sign reminds staff to engage latch before operating lift.

Source: INSIGHT IMAGING, Lake Forest, CA.

Figure 7-7. Visual Cues: Patient Positioning

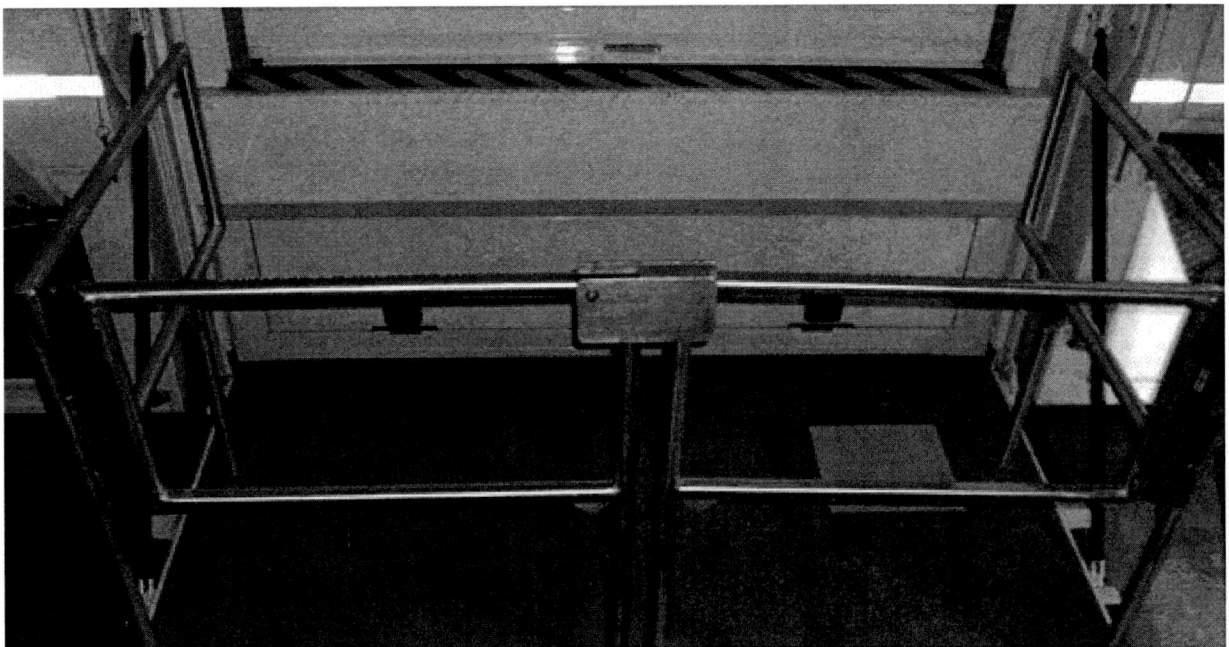

The yellow square (upper right-hand corner) was painted to designate where patients are to stand. The yellow tape strips in the railing in front of the square are where patients are to put their hands.

Source: INSIGHT IMAGING, Lake Forest, CA.

INDEX

Intraocular surgical instruments, cleaning and steriliz-
ing, 93, 94*t*
ISMP. *See* Institute for Safe Medication Practices
(ISMP)
IT. *See* Information technology (IT)

J

JC. *See* Joint Commission (JC)
JIT (just-in-time) approach, 102
Joint Commission (JC)
on anticoagulants, 34
Do Not Use List (prescription writing), 47, 49*f*
on fire safety, 114
on HAI prevention, 86
hand hygiene guidelines, 84, 85*t*
on laboratory testing, 19
on LASA medications, 43
on medication reconciliation, 44
on patient dentification, 5
on patient education, 7–8
on reducing MRI accidents and injuries, 97, 98*t*
standards
emergency preparedness, 93
infection control and prevention, 84
on surgical fires, 67
on surgical site infections, 67
survey on steam sterilization reprocessing, 95
on telephone reporting, 15
Universal Protocol for Preventing Wrong Site, Wrong
Procedure, and Wrong Person Surgery™, 68–
71
on verbal orders, 15
Just-in-time (JIT) approach, 102

K

Kaiser Permanente, 115
Kanban cards, 102

L

Labeling medication, 42–43
case study, 53–54
expiration date on multiuse vials, 42
risk reduction strategies, 43
Laboratory testing
errors in
causes, 22
factors contributing to, 22–23
follow-up in, 23, 24
imaging challenges and, 23
JC requirements for, 19

processes in, 20
case study, 26–31
error-free, 21*t*
management of, interventions to improve, 22*t*, 23
simple mapping, 21*t*, 23–25
Language. *See also* Communication
bilingualism and, 8
drug labeling, 9, 42
LASA medications. *See* Look-alike/sound-alike (LASA)
medications
Life Safety Code®, 91
Lift safety, mobile diagnostic/transport units, 113
case study, 122–126
Literacy
affect on patient's health care, 8–9
problems associated with, 9
Litigation, error disclosure and, 110
Look-alike/sound-alike (LASA) medications, 43–44
dispensing and storage, tips on, 44
JC requirements for, 43
visual controls for, 44

M

Magnetic resonance imaging (MRI)
accidents and injuries associated with, 97
JC recommendations and reduction strategies for,
97, 97*t*, 98*t*
mobile unit, lift safety in, 113
case study, 122–126
safety-risk identifiers for, 97
Malignant hyperthermia (MH)
case study, 72–73, 76–77
sample worksheets, 74*f*–75*f*
defined, 65
diagnostic tests for, 63
emergency therapy for, 64*f,* 65
event drill worksheet, 75*f*
susceptibility to, 65
Malignant Hyperthermia Association of the United
States, 65
sample worksheets, 74*f*–75*f*
Marking, operative site, 68–69, 71
Medical device malfunction, CT-induced, 99
Medication(s)
adverse events involving. *See* Medication errors
allergies to. *See* Medication allergies
card detailing patient's use, 47
labeling. *See* Labeling medication
look-alike/sound-alike. *See* Look-alike/sound-alike
(LASA) medications